SIRT FOOD DIET:

The Complete Guide to Lose Weight Fast, Burn Fat and Activate the Metabolism with Easy, Delicious and Healthy Recipes | 7-Day Meal Plan and Cookbook for Beginners.

Amy Stephens

Table of Contents

Introduction

Sirtfood Diet is a ground-breaking diet that gives the ability to turn on an old-fashioned family of genes that exists in every one of us. The name given to this family of genes is sirtuin. Sirtuins are unique since they orchestrate forms profound inside our cells that impact such significant things as our ability to burn fat, our susceptibility to illness, and even our life expectancy. Notable is the impact of sirtuins that they are currently alluded to as "master metabolic regulators." This is precisely what anybody needs to lose a few pounds and carry on with a long and healthy life.

Naturally, sirtuins have become the subject of extreme scientific research lately. The first sirtuin was found in 1984 in yeast and intrigued interest that genuinely took off through the span of the following three decades when it was uncovered that sirtuin activation improves life span, first in yeast, and afterward in mice.

From yeast to human beings and every other organism in the middle, the essential standards of cell metabolism are indistinguishable. If you can control something as modest as budding yeast and see an advantage, at that point, rehash it in higher living beings. For example, mice, the potential exists for similar benefits to be acknowledged in people.

Sirtuins are ancient families of genes with the ability to assist us with burning fat, form muscle, and keep us super healthy. It settled that sirtuins can be turned on through caloric limitation, fasting, and exercise; however, there is another progressive method to accomplish this: food. We consider the foods that generally aid in enacting sirtuins as Sirtfoods.

How sirtfood can help you lose weight

With the Sirtfood Diet, we have accomplished something exceptional. We've taken the most intense Sirtfoods on earth and have woven them into a fresh out of the box and better approach for eating, any semblance of which has never been seen. We have chosen the "most elite" from the most advantageous weight control diet at any point known and from them made a world-beating diet.

Without a doubt, one thing that may strike you from the list of Sirtfoods is their recognition. While you may not, right now, eat all the foods on the list, you in all probability are eating a few. So why are you not losing weight?

The appropriate response is discovered when we look at the changed components that the most forefront dietary science shows are required for building a diet that works. It's tied in with eating Sirtfoods in the correct amount, variety, and types. It's tied in with supplementing Sirtfood dishes with liberal servings of protein and afterward eating your meals at the best time. Also, it's about the opportunity to taste the genuinely delectable foods that you appreciate in the quantities you like.

The vast majority of us mostly don't consume almost enough Sirtfoods to inspire an intense fat-burning and health-boosting impact. When scientists looked at the utilization of five essential sirtuin-actuating supplements (quercetin, myricetin, kaempferol, luteolin, and apigenin) in the US diet, they saw singular everyday intake as scarcely 13 milligrams every day. Interestingly, standard Japanese admission was multiple times higher. Contrast that and our Sirtfood Diet enlightenment process, people will consume many milligrams of sirtuin-initiating supplements each day.

We are discussing a complete eating routine transformation where we increment our day by day admission of sirtuin-actuating supplements by as much as fiftyfold. While this may sound overwhelming or illogical, it truly isn't.

Juicing and Food

Juices and whole foods are indispensable to the Sirtfood Diet. Here, we are discussing extracts explicitly made utilizing a juicer—blenders and smoothie makers don't work. For some, this will appear to be irrational, on the premise that when something is juiced, the fiber is expelled. Yet, for leafy greens, this is actually what we need.

The fiber from food contains what are called non-extractable polyphenols (or NEPPs). These are polyphenols, including sirtuin activators, that are appended to the food's stringy piece and are possibly discharged when separated by our inviting stomach microbes. By expelling the fiber, we don't get the NEPPs and miss out on their integrity. Be that as it may, significantly, the NEPP content changes drastically, relying upon the kind of plant. The NEPP substance of foods like fruit, oats, and nuts is critical, and these oughts to be eaten entirely (in strawberries, NEPPs give more than 50 percent of the polyphenols!). Be that as it may, for leafy vegetables, the active ingredients in the Sirtfood juice are far lower despite a large, more significant part of the fiber.

So, with regards to leafy greens, we get the most extreme value for our money by juicing them and expelling the low-supplement fiber, which means we can utilize a lot more prominent volumes and accomplish a super concentrated hit of sirtuin-actuating polyphenols.

There is likewise another preferred position to expel the fiber. Leafy greens contain a kind of grain called insoluble fiber, which has a scouring activity in the stomach related structure. When we eat a lot of it, much the same as on the off chance that we over scrub something, it can aggravate and harm our stomach lining, that implies leafy green–stuffed smoothies will be fiber over-burden for some individuals, conceivably exasperating or in any event, causing IBS (irritable bowel syndrome) and ruining our assimilation of supplements.

Having a portion of your Sirtfoods in juice form can likewise have mostly favorable circumstances to retain their decency. For instance, one of the ingredients for the green juice is matcha green tea. When we consume the sirtuin activator, EGCG, found in elevated levels in green tea, in liquid form, its ingestion is 65 percent higher. We think that it's intriguing to note that when we ran blood tests on our own, changing from smoothies to green juices achieved increments of other fundamental supplements, such as magnesium and folic acid.

The crux is that to truly get those sirtuin genes reacting for emotional weight loss and health, we have to assemble a diet that consolidates the two juices and whole foods for the most extreme advantage.

The Quantity of Protein

Sirtfood meals ought to consistently be rich in or consist of a lot of proteins. A structural element of a dietary protein called Lucien has appeared to have extra advantages in invigorating SIRT1 to build fat-burning and improve glucose control.

Yet, Lucien also has another job, and this is the place its synergistic relationship with Sirtfoods truly counts. Lucien intensely stimulates anabolism in our cells, especially in muscle, which requests a great deal of energy and means our energy production structures (called mitochondria) need to stay at work longer than required. This makes a need in our cells for the movement of Sirtfoods. As you may review, one of the impacts of

Sirtfoods is to stimulate more mitochondria to be made, improve how effective they are, and make them burn fat as fuel. Subsequently, our bodies need them to fulfill this additional energy need. The given effect is that by combining Sirt Foods with dietary protein, we see a synergistic impact that supports sirtuin initiation and, at last, makes you burn fat to fuel muscle development and better health.

Fishes, especially oily ones, are an astoundingly decent protein source to supplement the activity of Sirtfoods, as they are rich in omega-3 unsaturated fats, notwithstanding their protein content. Without a doubt, you will have heard about the medical advantages of oily fish and explicitly omega-3 fish oils. Furthermore, presently late research proposes that the benefits of omega-3 fats may come through upgrading how our sirtuin genes work.

There have been concerns raised about the negative impacts of protein-rich diets on health as of late, and without Sirt Foods to offset the protein, we can start to get why. Lucien can be a double-edged blade. As we've stated, we need Sirtfoods to enable our cells to fulfill the metabolic need that Lucien puts on them. Be that as it may, without them, our mitochondria can get worn out, and as opposed to improving health, high Lucien levels can advance heftiness and insulin resistance. Sirtfoods help to keep the impacts of Lucien, under control as well as capably working in support of us. Consider Lucien juicing your foot on the quickening agent of weight loss and healthiness, with Sirtfoods the apparatus that guarantees the cell satisfies the expanded need.

Eat Early

Regarding eating, our way of thinking is before the better, in a perfect world, completing the process of eating for the day by 7 p.m. This is for two reasons. In the first place, to harvest the characteristic satisfying impact of Sirtfoods. There's significantly more advantage to eating a meal that will keep you feeling full, fulfilled, and stimulated as you approach your day rather than spend the entire day exploring hungry just to eat and remain full as you stay asleep from sundown to sunset.

There is a second convincing explanation: to continue dietary patterns on top of your inner body clock. As a whole, we have worked in a body clock called our circadian rhythm, which manages a considerable lot of our standard body abilities as indicated by the hour of the day. In addition to other things, it impacts how the body handles the food we eat. The body's clockwork in synchrony, basically following the signals of the light-dark pattern of the sun. As diurnal organisms, we're intended to be dynamic in the daytime as opposed to during the darkness of the night. Thus, our body clock gears us up to deal with food most productively during the day, when it is light, and we are relied upon to be dynamic, and less so when it is nighttime, where we are somewhat prepared for rest and sleep.

The issue is that many of us have "work clocks" and "social clocks" that are not in a state of harmony with the setting of the sun. At night, in some cases, there is no possibility that a few of us get the chance to eat. To a certain extent, we can prepare our body clock to match up to various calendars, such as "evening chronotypes" who like or must be dynamic, eat, and rest later in the day. In any case, living that does not align with the outer light-dark cycle holds some significant disadvantages. Studies find that night chronotype people have expanded susceptibility to accumulate fat, muscle loss, and metabolic issues, just as regularly experiencing inadequate rest. This is actually what we see among people that work night shifts, who have a higher chance of gaining weight and metabolic disorders, which is at any rate halfway because of the impacts of their late eating schedule.

The result is that you're in an ideal situation eating prior in the day whenever the situation allows, in a perfect world by 7 p.m. Be that as it may, imagine a scenario where this is simply not possible. Fortunately, sirtuins assume a crucial job in body clock synchronization.

Chapter 1: What is Sirtfood Diet

The Sirtfood Diet is initially created and named by Masters in Nutritional Medicine, Aiden Goggins, and Glen Matten.

Initially, their goal was to find a healthier way for people to eat but, when they did a trial of their program, people started shedding weight rapidly. Considering the millions of people around the world who are struggling to lose a single pound, it would have been incredibly selfish if this health plan was not shared with the world. Most of the initial research group participants lost an average of 7 pounds in 7 days (Happening, 2016).

The plan that these men developed focuses on combining certain foods, eaten in a way to maximize the delivery of nutrition to our body. It incorporates an initial, minimal stage of restricting calories to give your body a period to reset and eliminate some of the built-up waste that is damaging your body. This is followed by a maintenance phase to help you acclimatize to the new foods you're eating and, ideally, set you up for life-long success. During all the stages, you will incorporate powerful green juices and well-structured, well-planned meals.

The diet is centered around so-called "sirtfoods," which are plant-based foods that are known to activate a gene in the human body called a sirtuin. Sirtuins belong to an entire family of proteins, labeled SIRT1 through to SIRT7, and each has unique connections to health. These proteins help insulate and protect our cells from inflammation and other damage from daily operations, helping to reduce our risk of developing major diseases, especially those related to aging.

Studies have shown that when people eat diets rich in these sirtuin-activating foods, they live longer, healthier, free from diabetes, heart disease, and even dementia. You may be interested in the diet for its weight-loss potential, but it turns out that healthy body composition is a natural by-product of good health.

Unfortunately, most Americans eat a diet that is notably lacking in sirtfoods, which presents a clear connection to our culture of disease and dysfunctional aging.

The Sirtfood Diet is not a miracle cure or even a one-week program designed to get you wedding-ready. If you're only interested in losing a few pounds so you can take some photos for your social media accounts and then return to your old habits, there may be other diets or programs that will better suit your needs.

The Sirtfood Diet is a blueprint to help guide you through the rest of your life, choosing delicious foods that will not just impress your taste buds but also enhance nearly every aspect of your health. If you switch from a Standard American Diet (SAD) to the diet and lifestyle, you will lose any weight that your body doesn't need.

A healthy body doesn't store extra energy. It asks for what it needs, and it uses it effectively.

The diet isn't designed to encourage you to starve or deprive yourself. The fact is that the designer made it to deny you foods that are deficient of nutrients, and, even though they have many calories, your cells still starve for nutrition, in order to to help you thrive. The Sirtfood Diet is the opposite of deprivation and starvation. It is nourishment and balance.

The foods you'll incorporate during the first two stages of the diet are mainly from the Top 20 Sirtfoods. Once you're adapted to these core foods, you can add in many other nutrient-rich foods. In Appendix 2, there is a list of 100 foods rich in polyphenols, which are also effective sirtuin-activating compounds (STACs).

Most people following the SAD may use 20 ingredients in a month, let alone enjoy the sheer volume of choice ingredients from the 120 options you will learn about.

In recent decades, an alarming number of people have concluded that healthy food is boring, and plants, specifically vegetables, are terrible tasting. This is because the foods we've become dependant on – packed with sugar, salt, and unhealthy fats – have chemically altered our connection to food. Our brains are mostly lying to us, and our taste buds have been compromised.

This is one of the reasons the week-long reset is so necessary. After this first week, you will be able to taste food differently. The more times you expose yourself to the plant-based foods suggested, the more enjoyment you will get out of them.

That being said, you probably already genuinely enjoy many of the options on the Top 20 list, such as strawberries, olive oil, red onions, blueberries and, of course, I can't forget coffee, chocolate, and red wine. The shopping list doesn't sound too terrible, now does it?

Why Choose Sirtfoods

Sirtfoods are simply the name given to foods that activate the human body's sirtuin gene. Everyone has sirtuins; however, not everyone's body is well adapted to getting the most out of their genes.

Sirtuins regulate many critical functions related closely to our body weight and metabolic system, including our ability to burn fat and build muscle. They've also been shown to be a compelling force in aging and developing a disease, notably, reducing risk factors for both conditions (Happening, 2016).

We want to be able to turn these genes on so that we can protect our cells, and enjoying a life-long diet rich in sirt foods is one of the most effective ways to make this happen.

Sirtfoods do more than just activate a gene, however. There are many reasons for you to adopt a sirtfood lifestyle, and they are all health-focused.

The Standard American Diet (SAD), on the other hand, is a way of life that is more consistently disease-focused. Characterized by large quantities of red meat and processed meats, pre-packaged foods, vegetable oils, refined grains, and a lot of sugar, there is a distinct and almost total lack of micronutrition.

Macronutrients, carbohydrates, fats, and proteins provide our bodies with energy. They establish a standard measurement of calories consumed.

Micronutrients, such as vitamins, minerals, fiber, antioxidants, and phytonutrients, are supposed to come with our calories, but in the SAD, they are in minimal supply.

It is no secret that plants offer the most nutrition per calorie consumed. Every edible plant has a unique nutritional profile that provides your body with an exclusive range of benefits. This is why having a lot of variety in the types of plants you eat will better protect you from an innumerable variety of illnesses.

When you decide not to stop actively damaging your body, but start providing the natural nutrition your body needs to heal, our bodies are fantastically resilient. The human body has built-in disease-fighting biological systems. All they need to protect us is the right food source to keep them going.

Sirtfoods, and other plant-based sources of nutrition, give your body what it needs to stay young, disease-free, and at an ideal weight.

The Sirtfood Diet is more than just a list of high foods, though. It's designed to give you a system for combining these foods in the most effective way to help your body get the most out of the nutrition you provide.

Nutrition is not a pill; you can pop to excuse an otherwise unhealthy lifestyle. Studies have repeatedly shown us that many vitamins, minerals, and other highly nutritious compounds aren't properly absorbed by our body when they are isolated and converted into a supplement or pill.

Imagine each food item is a recipe. If you follow the method correctly, you will end up with perfectly baked lasagna. If you try to isolate the essence of lasagna down to a single ingredient, you will end up with boring pasta noodles, or greasy, baked cheese, or possibly just some oregano, but you will not have lasagna.

The same can be said for whole foods. If you isolate a single antioxidant from blueberry and put it in a pill, your body will be as unimpressed as you would be if you served a plate of boiled pasta.

The world of medical science is advancing at such a fast pace, it's mesmerizing and inspiring. But we still do not fully understand how our amazing complex biological systems break down and utilize the equally complex nutrition that comes from the food we eat. But we do know that plenty of whole, plant-based foods can, quite literally, save your life.

Chapter 2: What is Sirtuins?

Sirtuins, or SIRT for short, belong to the family of proteins that regulate cell health, including homeostasis. Hemostasis is the process by which the body maintains its stability and adjusts the conditions most conducive to its survival. The SIRT family of proteins includes seven members (SIRT1-7). The yeast mute information regulator SIR2 is the founding member of the SIRT family of proteins, which controls chromatin, DNA recombination, and gene expression. Among the seven mammalian SIRTs, SIRT1, SIRT2, and SIRT3 have a deacetylase capacity. The other remaining SIRTs (SIRT4, SIRT5, SIRT6, and SIRT7) have weak or undetectable deacetylate activity. SIRT1-7 differ in their function and location.

SIRT1 is located in the cytosol and in the cell nucleus, where it fulfills its cell life function. It is involved in glucose metabolism, neurodegeneration, differentiation, control of gene expression, aging, cell death, and tumor development. SIRT2 is in the cytosol and catalyzes the deacetylation of alpha-tubulin (Lys40), H31ys56, FOXO1, H41ys16, and FOXO3a. It also involves gene expression regulation, tubulin acetylation, tubulin acetylation, cell cycle regulation, response to DNA damage, cancer, and neurodegeneration... Localization of SIRT3 on the inner membrane of the mitochondria with long-chain substrates acyl-CoA dehydrogenase (LCDA), acetyl-CoA synthetase 2 (ACS2), 2,3-hydroxy-3-methyl glutaryl CoA synthetase 2 (HMGCS2), ornithine Transcarbamoyl transferase (OTC), glutamate dehydrogenase (GDH), cycle-Philip D, superoxide dismutase 2 (SOD2), Isocitrate dehydrogenase 2 (IDH2), many components of the respiratory chain complexes of mitochondria and Ku70. It is responsible for the production of mitochondrial ATP, the oxidation of fatty acids, and the regulation of mitochondrial protein. It also controls caloric restriction and cellular response to oxidative stress by activating SOD2 and IDH2, which reduces oxidized reactive oxygen species (ROS) and glutathione. It is also involved in the suppression of tumors and cell death, which has a positive impact on genomic stability. SIRT4 is in the mitochondrial matrix. It is engaged in the ribosylation of ADP and inhibition of GHD using NAD +. SIRT5 is also found in the mitochondrial matrix and contains a decarboxylase dependent on NAD + and the desuccinylase activity in CPS1.

SIRT6, which acts as a deacetylase and ADP ribosyltransferase, is necessary for telomeric functions, hemostasis of metabolism, DNA repair, and genome stability. SIRT7 is mainly a nucleolar protein that regulates the transcription of ribosomal genes by interaction with RNA polymerase 1. SIRT7 has a high selectivity for H31ys18 and a deacetylase dependent on NAD +. When SIRT7 is deacetylated, we must suppress the genes involved in cell anchoring and inhibit contact, promoting the malignant phenotype of tumor cells. As well as desuccinylase activity in CPS1. SIRT6, which acts as a deacetylase and ADP ribosyltransferase, is necessary for the functions of telomeres, hemostasis of metabolism, DNA repair, and genome stability. SIRT7 is mainly a nucleolar protein that regulates the transcription of ribosomal genes by interaction with RNA polymerase 1.

SIRT7 has a high selectivity for H31ys18 and a deacetylase dependent on NAD +. When SIRT7 is deacetylated, we need to suppress the genes involved in cell anchoring and inhibit contact, thus promoting tumor cells' malignant phenotype. As well as the desuccinylase activity in CPS1. SIRT6, which acts as a deacetylase and ADP ribosyltransferase, is necessary for telomeric functions, hemostasis of metabolism, DNA repair, and genome stability. SIRT7 is mainly a nucleolar protein that regulates the transcription of ribosomal genes through interaction with RNA polymerase 1. SIRT7 has a high selectivity for H31ys18 and a deacetylase dependent on NAD +. When SIRT7 is deacetylating, we must suppress the genes involved in cell anchoring and inhibit contact, promoting the malignant phenotype of tumor cells.

Genome stability. SIRT7 is mainly a nucleolar protein that regulates the transcription of ribosomal genes by interaction with RNA polymerase 1. SIRT7 has a high selectivity for H31ys18 and a deacetylase dependent on NAD +. When SIRT7 is deacetylated, we need to suppress the genes involved in cell anchoring and inhibit contact, thus promoting tumor cells' malignant phenotype. Genome stability. SIRT7 is mainly a nucleolar protein that regulates the transcription of ribosomal

17

genes by interaction with RNA polymerase 1. SIRT7 has a high selectivity for H31ys18 and a deacetylase dependent on NAD +. When SIRT7 is deacetylating, we need to suppress the genes involved in cell anchoring and inhibit contact, thus promoting tumor cells' malignant phenotype.

The science of sirt food

The sirt diet cannot be classified as low in carbohydrates or low in fat. This diet is very different from its many predecessors and, at the same time, advocates many of the same things: eating fresh plant foods. As the name suggests, it is a diet based on sirtuins. But what are sirtuins, and why have you never heard of them?

There are seven Sirtuin proteins: SIRT-1 to SIRT-7a. They can be found in all cells and the cells of all animals on the planet. Sirtuins are found in almost all living organisms and nearly all parts of the cell and control what happens. The supplement company Elysium Health compares body cells to an office with sirtuins, which act as CEOs and help cells respond to internal and external changes. They regulate what is done when it has done and who does it.

Of the seven sirtuins, one acts in the cytoplasm of your cell, three in the mitochondria of the cell, and three in the cell nucleus. They are busy, but they mainly eliminate acetyl groups from other proteins. These acetyl groups indicate that the protein to which they are attached is available to perform its function. The sirtuins remove the available flag and prepare the protein for use.

Sirtuins seem quite crucial for the normal functioning of your body. Why have you never heard of it?

The first sirtuin discovered was SIR2, a gene found in the 1970s that controlled fruit flies' ability to mate. It wasn't until the 1990s that scientists discovered other similar proteins in almost all forms of life. Each organism had a different amount of sirtuins: bacteria have one, and yeast has five. Experiments on mice show that they have the same number as humans, seven.

Sirtuins have been shown to prolong the life of yeasts and mice. So far, there is no evidence of the same effect in humans, but these sirtuins are present in almost all forms of life, and many scientists hope that organisms as distant as yeast and mice will have the same effect as sirtuins. Activation can also be extended to humans.

In addition to sirtuins, our body needs another substance called.

Nicotinamide adenine dinucleotide for cells to function correctly. Elysium (see above) compares this substance to the money a business needs to keep it going. Like any CEO, a sirtuin can only manage the business properly if there is sufficient cash flow. NAD + was first discovered in 1906. You get your diet from NAD + from your diet by eating foods made from the building blocks of NAD +.

Other benefits of sirtuin

By actuating our old sirtuin genes, we can burn fat and construct a more slender and healthy body. What's more, with sirtuins at the center of our metabolism and their significance stretches out a long way past body components alone, to each feature of our healthiness.

Think about an ailment that you partner with getting old, and the odds are an absence of sirtuin movement in the body is included. For instance, sirtuin initiation is extraordinary for heart health, securing the heart's muscle cells and, for the most part, helping the heart work better. It likewise improves how our bodies work, causes us to handle cholesterol all the more proficiently and secures against the stopping up of our veins and arteries known as atherosclerosis.

Sirtuin enactment expands the measure of insulin that can be discharged and causes it to work all the more successfully in the body. As it occurs, one of the most famous antidiabetic drugs, metformin, depends on SIRT1 for its valuable impact. To be sure, one pharmaceutical organization is currently exploring adding sirtuin activators to metformin treatment for diabetics, with results from creatures demonstrating a fantastic 83 percent decrease in the portion of metformin required for similar impacts.

With regards to the brain, sirtuins are included once more, with the sirtuin movement lower in Alzheimer's patients.

Interestingly, sirtuin activation improves correspondence flags in the cerebrum, upgrades intellectual ability, and lessens mind aggravation. This stops the development of amyloid-β creation and tau protein accumulation, two of the fundamental harming things we see happening in Alzheimer's patients' cerebrums.

Osteoblasts are exceptional cells in our bones responsible for building new bone. The more osteoblasts we have, the stronger our bones. Sirtuin enactment advances the creation of osteoblast cells, yet also, it builds their endurance. This makes sirtuin initiation essential for long-lasting bone health.

Malignant growth has been a progressively dubious region for sirtuin studies. Keeping in mind that ongoing examination shows that sirtuin enactment assists with stifling disease tumors, researchers are just barely starting to disentangle this intricate field. While there is considerably more to learn on this specific point, those societies that eat the most Sirtfood Have the least malignancy rates, as we will before long observe.

Heart diseases, diabetes, dementia, osteoporosis, and likely cancer: it's a noteworthy list of infections that can be forestalled by initiating sirtuins. It might not shock discover that societies eating a lot of Sirtfoods as a significant aspect of their current weight control plans experience a life span and healthiness a large portion of us could scarcely envision. You'll hear more very soon.

That leaves us with an energizing end: basically by including the world's most intense Sirtfoods to your diet and making that a deep-rooted propensity. You also can encounter this degree of healthiness's only the tip of the iceberg—all while getting the build you need.

Chapter 3: How Sirt Foods Help Burn Fat

Burn Fat

In addition to protecting your muscles, sirtfoods encourage your metabolic system to start burning through the fat stored in your body, which is one of the reasons for the extraordinary weight loss potential.

Gaining weight is a complex process for humans that involves multiple hormones sending signals back and forth to your various biological processes. One of these hormones, insulin, I'm sure you're familiar with.

When you consume any calories, your body needs to convert the food into glucose so that it can be used as energy to keep your body functioning. Some foods, such as sugar or refined carbohydrates, convert to sugar in your bloodstream almost instantaneously, causing a spike in blood glucose levels.

Like complex carbohydrates and proteins, other foods take longer for your body to break down and convert to glucose, so your blood gets a more slow and steady drip of glucose.

When your blood sugar gets too high because you've consumed more sugar than your body needs to operate immediately, it can cause various problems. Headaches, thirst, or fatigue might be experienced in the short-term, but high blood sugar levels can lead to kidney failure, heart disease, or nerve damage if the issue becomes chronic.

These symptoms are severe and potentially life-threatening, so your body has a process to detect high blood sugar levels and bring them back down: it releases insulin.

With the help of your liver and cholesterol, insulin pulls sugar out of your bloodstream and tells your cells to take it instead, and your blood glucose levels drop as your fat cells get a little more full.

When your blood sugar gets too low, another hormone, glucagon, will be released. Glucagon taps your liver and fat cells to release the stored glucose back into your bloodstream.

The main problem with our modern diet is that humans have developed the habit of constant grazing and over-eating. This provides a continuous flow of glucose, triggering a constant need for insulin. Our blood sugar rarely dips low enough to trigger glucagon production, so instead of using our stored energy, we add more to the reserves.

Swapping a Standard American Diet (SAD) that causes an instant spike in your blood glucose for a Sirtfood Diet, which will create a more slow and steady flow of energy will help to reinstate that natural balance of hormones once again. As a bonus, studies have shown that activating sirtuins can suppress your body's ability to store fat as it increases the propensity to burn it (Picard et al., 2004). Your metabolic system will have a chance to use the stored energy.

Aside from sirtfoods being a more balancing form of energy, our cells are being protected and fortified by activating our sirtuin genes. Each cell has a power center called a mitochondrion responsible for converting glucose into usable energy. This is a lot of work for our cells. Especially if we are eating more calories than we need and those calories are primarily simple carbohydrates, our mitochondria wear out quickly.

Sirtuins protect our mitochondria, allowing them to process energy more efficiently. In other words, we can burn fat more quickly.

Sirtfoods work on multiple fronts to help our body naturally regulate weight: they reduce the amount of glucose that gets stored as fat, increasing the speed at which our fat gets used.

As a bonus, by naturally regulating our metabolism, we can protect ourselves against insulin resistance and type 2 diabetes.

Insulin and glycogen aren't the only hormones to return to a healthy balance on a Sirtfood Diet. Leptin is also regulated.

Leptin resistance isn't as commonly understood as insulin resistance, but it plays just as crucial of a role in the process of weight gain. Leptin is often called the hunger hormone because it's responsible for telling your brain when you have enough fat stored in your body to keep you safe, and when you need to take in more energy.

If you have low body fat, your brain will throw out hunger signals to encourage you to eat more food. Unfortunately, if you have damaged leptin receptors, your mind will also continue to pump out hunger signals, whether you're actually in need of energy or not.

Hunger is very hard to ignore. If your leptin levels are dysregulated, not only are you going to always feel hungry, but your body will also be actively trying to store any energy you consume as fat instead of using it immediately.

When you follow a Sirtfood Diet, your leptin levels will naturally balance, and your hunger signals will start to spark when you genuinely need more nutrition, not merely when your sugar crash has taken a turn for the worse.

When all the hormones associated with your metabolism are operating and communicating effectively, you will only store as much body fat as necessary. If you're currently overweight, repairing your metabolic system will help you quickly release weight until you reach your optimal body composition.

How It Works (how to lose 3.5 lbs. in just seven days)

The first seven days are the most difficult, as you can consume a maximum of 1000 calories per day in the early three days, then

1500 calories from day 3 to day 7. The menus are based on smoothies and centrifuged vegetables (the so-called green juices) in the first three days, with only one substantial meal of your choice, but always based on Sirt food cooked with ad-hoc preparation (a light development may still be excellent). From day four, with an additional 500 calories, you can add substantial meals. In the first week, the Diet Sirt allows you to lose just over 3 kg.

The second phase goes from the 8th to the 21st day and includes three solid meals a day, plenty of Sirt food (but I remain in a range of 2000kcal), and a green juice based on Sirt vegetables.

Here is the preparation of centrifuged green juice. The green extract can purify, satiate, and be the protagonist of the first week of the food plan.

To prepare it, it takes:

· 75 g kale

· 30 g arugula

· 5 g parsley

· 150 g green celery with leaves

· 1/2 green apple

· 1/2 lemon juice

· 1/2 teaspoon satin matcha teaspoon

Preparation Centrifuge

the kale, rocket, and parsley; add celery and grated apple; enrich with half a squeezed lemon and half teaspoon of matcha tea. Drink immediately so as not to lose the beneficial effects of vegetables and not to store it in the fridge. It must always be prepared at the time of consumption.

The green juice should be consumed half an hour before breakfast, lunch, and dinner and possibly never eat more than 7 p.m.

Sirtfoods and their nutrients

While all plants have these pressure reaction structures, just certain ones have been created to deliver significant measures of sirtuin-enacting polyphenols. We call these plants Sirtfoods. Their disclosure implies that rather than fasting or laborious exercise programs, there is presently a progressive better approach to initiate your sirtuin genes: eating a diet with adequate Sirtfoods.

It's so flawlessly straightforward, so natural, and this is how nature proposed us to eat, instead of the stomach rumbling or calorie tallying of present-day slimming down. Recall this: the cutting edge way to deal with diet is just 150 years of age; Sirtfoods were created naturally more than a billion years prior.

Furthermore, with that, you're presumably tingling to comprehend what explicit foods consider Sirtfoods. So right away, here are the best twenty Sirt Foods and their nutrients:

SIRTFOOD	NUTRIENT
Arugula	Quercetin, kaempferol
Chilies	Luteolin, myricetin
Buckwheat	Rutin
Capers	Kaempferol, quercetin
Celery	Apigenin, luteolin
Cocoa	Epicatechin
Coffee	Caffeic acid
Extra virgin olive oil	Oleuropein, hydroxytyrosol
Garlic	Ajoene, myricetin
Green tea	Epigallocatechin gallate (EGCG)
Kale	Kaempferol, quercetin
Medjool dates	Gallic acid, caffeic acid
Parsley	Apigenin, myricetin
Red endive	Luteolin
Red onion	Quercetin
Red wine	Resveratrol, piceatannol
Soy	Daidzein, formononetin
Strawberries	Fisetin
Turmeric	Curcumin

Walnuts	Gallic acid
Buckwheat	Rutin
Capers	Kaempferol, quercetin
Celery	Apigenin, luteolin
Cocoa	Epicatechin
Coffee	Caffeic acid
Extra virgin olive oil	Oleuropein, hydroxytyrosol
Garlic	Ajoene, myricetin
Green tea	Epigallocatechin gallate (EGCG)
Kale	Kaempferol, quercetin
Medjool dates	Gallic acid, caffeic acid
Parsley	Apigenin, myricetin
Red endive	Luteolin
Red onion	Quercetin
Red wine	Resveratrol, piceatannol
Soy	Daidzein, formononetin
Strawberries	Fisetin
Turmeric	Curcumin
Walnuts	Gallic acid

Sirt foods VS Fasting

This leads us to a big question: if sirtuin activation increases muscle mass, why do we lose muscle when we fast? After all, fasting activates our sirtuin genes as well. And herein lies one of the massive drawbacks of fasting.

This leads to a big question: if activation of the sirtuin increases muscle mass, why do we lose muscle when we fast? Fasting also stimulates our sirtuin genes, after all. And therein lies one of the fasting 's significant drawbacks.

Bear with us as we dig through the workings of this. Not all skeletal muscles are created equal to each other. We have two principal forms, called type-1 and type-2 conveniently. Type-1 tissue is used for longer length movements, while the type-2 muscle is used for brief bursts of more vigorous activity. And here's where it gets intriguing: fasting increases SIRT1 activity only in type-1 muscle fibers, not type-2. But type-1 muscle fiber size is preserved and even significantly increases when we fast.8 Unfortunately, in complete contrast to what happens in type-1 fibers during fasting, SIRT1 decreases rapidly in type-2 fibers. It means that fat burning slows down, and muscle breaks down to provide heat, instead.

But fasting for the muscles is a double-edged sword, with our type-2 fibers taking a hit. Type-2 fibers form the bulk of our concept of muscle. And even though our type-1 fiber mass is growing, with fasting, we also see a substantial overall loss of muscle. If we were able to avoid the breakdown, it would make us look aesthetically good and encourage more loss of weight. And the way to do this is to combat the decrease in SIRT1 in muscle fiber type-2 that is caused by fasting.

Researchers at Harvard Medical School tested this in an elegant mice study. They found that the signals for muscle breakdown were turned off, and no muscle loss occurred by stimulating SIRT1 activity in type-2 fibers during fasting.

The researchers then went a step further and tested the effects of increased SIRT1 activity on the muscle when the mice were fed rather than fasted, and found it stimulated very rapid growth of the muscle. In a week, muscle fibers with elevated SIRT1 activity displayed an impressive weight gain of 20 percent.

Such results are very close to the outcome of our Sirtfood Diet trial, but in turn, our research has been milder. After increasing SIRT1 activity after consuming a diet rich in sirtfoods, most participants had no muscle loss — and for others, it was only a moderately strong, muscle mass that increased.

Chapter 4: The Procedure of Sirtfood Diet

After you've filled your head with more molecular biological information that you probably needed in high school or college, let's take a look at the following steps on how to follow the diet and fill your fridge.

It is effortless to start the sirt food diet. It only takes a little preparation. If you don't know what kale is or where you can find green tea, you may have a learning curve, albeit a tiny one. There are a few ways to start the sirt diet.

While you prepare and cook healthy food, you may want to do a few things over:

1. Clean your cupboards and refrigerator of foods that are unhealthy and might tempt you. They also have a deficient calorie intake, and you don't want to be tempted to find a quick fix that could slow you down. Even if you have new recipes, you may think your old comfort foods are now more comfortable.

2. Buy all the ingredients you need for the week. If you buy what you need, it's more profitable. Once you see the recipes, you will notice that there are many overlapping ingredients. You will know your portions when dieting, but at least you have what you need, and you will save yourself a few trips to the store.

3. Wash, dry, cut, and store all the food you need to quickly prepare it when you need it. This will make a new diet less annoying.

A necessary kitchen tool that you need in addition to real food is a juicer. You will need a juicer as soon as the sirt diet begins. Centrifuges are everywhere, so they're relatively easy to find, but the quality varies a lot. This is where price, function, and comfort come in. You can go to a famous department store or find them online. Once you know what you are looking for, you can look around.

The extractor's quality determines the nutritional quality and, sometimes, the taste of its juice, which we will explain below. You need to know that buying a cheap juicer is a good idea now. However, if you choose to upgrade later, you will have spent more money twice. When you buy a good juicer, consider it an investment in your health. Many people have paid money to become a member of a gym that has not quadrupled the cost of a juicer. A juicer is not wasted.

Since not all juicers are created equal, let's list some of the features you want to look for.

How to Make the Sirtfood Plan

You may have heard of the Sirtfood plan before, especially since singer Adele reportedly lost 50 pounds after the program, but do you know what it is? The nutrition plan defines the 20 foods that activate the so-called "lean genes," increasing your metabolism and energy levels. He even claims that he could lose 7 kg in 7 days. The diet plan changes the way you eat healthily. It may sound like a not accessible name, but you will hear a lot about it. Since the "Sirt" in Sirt Foods is a shortcut for sirtuin genes, a group of genes nicknamed "skinny genes" that, frankly, work like magic.

Eating these foods, plan makers, nutritionists Aidan Goggins and Glen Matten, activate these genes and "mimic the effects of calorie constraint, fasting, and exercise." It enables a recycling process in the body, "which removes cellular debris and the condition that builds up over time and causes health problems and loss of vitality," the authors write.

Tips for Success

Burns fat strengthens muscles and improves cellular physical condition: these are the guaranteed results of the SirtFood diet.

Being healthy and losing weight is a daily option. You need to take these first steps to see how it can change you and your life.

If you want to get fantastic results from SirtFoods, here are some suggestions on how to start your diet:

Safety first- Before starting a particular food or treatment, contact your doctor, especially if you have an existing illness. This ensures that the eating does not sabotage any medications that you are taking or that are harmful to your health. Don't worry; the SirtFood diet is pretty safe.

Knowledge is power- This diet is still new, but there is always the right amount of information and closer because it is rapidly gaining popularity. You can also search the Internet for recipes, food alternatives, nutrient levels, and much more.

Follow the directions - SirtFood guarantees results if you follow the recommended nutritional guidelines and foods precisely.

Help yourself- In addition to the diet program instructions, you can first remove processed and starchy foods from your healthy diet. Stop eating garbage! This will speed up the results of the SirtFood diet.

Start physical activity- The SirtFood diet can burn these fats and build muscle, but I recommend adding physical activity to your daily routine. Walking for 30 minutes a day would do wonders for your body and also speed up the results. Also, there are many incredible effects of training, e.g., preventing and fighting health problems, improving mood, promoting better sleep, burning calories, boosting energy, and much more.

Go to the supermarket- The SirtFood diet depends on certain foods. These foods have been selected for their ability to activate sirtuins. So if you don't follow the list, you won't see any results. Don't worry, and I will provide you with a list of recommended foods. Also, there are no overpriced foods, and you can find them almost anywhere (there may even be something hiding in your fridge).

Be prepared with the initial "restrictions"- If you want to obtain different results, you have to "sacrifice" a little to benefit from all the benefits of the SirtFood diet. Don't worry, though, the first three days are the hardest for this diet as there are calorie restrictions, but rest assured that it gets easier every day. Although the restrictions imposed were not as severe for those who tried the diet, the reason was careful planning of meals. You will not be hungry with this diet if you choose wisely.

Plan your meals- Whatever your diet, planning your meals is helpful. This reduces the stress of eating and gives you the ability to weigh your selection and fill your cupboard. For the first phase of this diet you need to do a calorie count. You will be amazed that there are many dishes with fewer calories and plenty of sirtuins.

Hire a dietary partner- This diet can also benefit your family, partner, or friends (not only those who are overweight). It's also more comfortable if you have a responsible partner who calls you back, shares recipes, or even cooks dishes.

Document your progress- You can start by taking "before" photos and make the required body measurements. You can also keep a food diary to track your food intake. Watch the changes in your body every week or phase. You can also have several goals to encourage him further to continue the diet.

Be careful to yourself- Don't set too many expectations. Yes, some can quickly lose 7 pounds in a week, but keep in mind that not all of our bodies are the same; And of course, your commitment counts. Other variables could be adding a workout plan to the diet plan, which could speed up the weight loss process.

Common mistakes to avoid professionals:

"Sirt foods" apparently trigger sirtuin in your body, a type of protein that protects your cells from death and contact disease and also controls your body's metabolism.

Forty gym participants found that each one lost an average of 7 pounds per week without losing muscle weight.

You can eat reasonable amounts of dark chocolate and wine all the time without being affected.

These are mostly healthy and nutritious foods like blueberries, nuts, and green tea.

It is useful in the long term and makes it healthy for life while reducing the aging process.

Sirtfood for building muscle

Sirtuins are a group of proteins with different effects. Sirt-1 is the protein responsible for causing the body to burn fat rather than muscle for energy, which is a miracle for weight loss. Another useful aspect of Sirt-1 is its ability to improve skeletal muscle.

Skeletal muscle is all the muscles you voluntarily control, such as the muscles in your limbs, back, shoulders, and so on. There are two other types; cardiac muscle is what the heart is formed of, while the smooth muscle is your involuntary muscles – which includes muscles around your blood vessels, face, and various parts of organs and other tissues.

Skeletal muscle is separated into two different groups, the blandly named type-1, and type-2. Type 1 muscle is effective at continued, sustained activity, whereas type-2 muscle is effective at short, intense periods of activity. For example, you would predominantly use type-1 muscles for jogging, but type-2 muscles for sprinting.

Sirt-1 protects the type-1 muscles, but not the type-2 muscle, which is still broken down for energy. Therefore, holistic muscle mass drops when fasting, even though type-1 skeletal muscle mass increases.

Sirt-1 also influences how the muscles work. Sirt-1 is produced by the muscle cells, but the ability to produce Sirt-1 decreases as the muscle ages. As a result, muscle is harder to build as you age and doesn't grow as fast in response to exercise. A lack of sirt-1 also causes the muscles to become tired quicker and gradually decline over time.

When you consider these effects of Sirt-1, you can start to form a picture of why fasting helps keep the body supple. Fasting releases Sirt-1, which in turn helps skeletal muscle grow and stay in good shape. Sirt-1 is also released by consuming sirtuin activators, giving the sirtfood diet its muscle retaining power.

Chapter 5: Sirt Food Ingredients

Sirtfoods are plant-based foods that activate a sirtuin. Sirtuins belong to a family of proteins that help insulate and protect our cells from damage, reducing our risk of developing any or all major diseases.

Many people turn to diets as a means of losing weight, and the Sirtfood Diet has been proven to be very good at helping achieve this goal. However, the interesting finding is that the diet isn't a weight management tool, so much as a strategy for enhancing overall health to live longer, healthier lives, free from diabetes, heart disease, and even dementia. It only turns out that healthy body weight is a natural by-product of good health.

Unfortunately, the Standard American Diet (SAD), also sometimes referred to as the Western Pattern Diet (WPD), is notably lacking in sirtfoods. There is a distinct and clear connection between our culture of disease and dysfunctional eating.

I'll introduce you to a list of the Top 20 Sirtfoods, which are featured prominently in all of the recipes in this book. I've also included a supplementary list of ten fruits and ten vegetables that are also very rich in sirtuin-activators and common throughout these recipes.

You'll notice that the vast majority of the ingredients are already commonly used and enjoyed, especially if you already cook some or most of your meals at home.

This makes the recipes feel somewhat familiar and achievable, but by sticking to the top sirtfoods, it makes shopping convenient and easy. You'll get to know the ingredients quickly, develop your confidence for tweaking recipes, and build your unique versions.

Healthy, home cooked food should never be boring or distasteful, and they don't have to be difficult either. Plants have such an incredible array of flavors and aromas that you'll find your sirtfood meals exciting and packed with just as much flavor as nutrition.

Get the right ingredients

Remember that all this diet asks from you is to increase your sirtuins intake. That can be done only through careful and selective grocery shopping. Prepare a list of the ingredients that contain a high amount of sirtuins and check their utility as per your meal plan. There are certain ingredients like coffee, parsley, red wine, and chocolate, that you can have all the time. So, stock up your kitchen cabinets with these ingredients.

Set up the schedule

The sirtfood diet gives you small weight loss targets for each week. In the initial time period, you must prepare a schedule to keep track of your meals, the caloric intake, and the timing of green juices you are consuming in a day. In this way, you will be able to manage the first few days of the diet adoption easily and continue observing body changes and measure your weight to keep track of your pace.

Prepare for the first week

In the first week of the sirtfood diet, the dieter must control his caloric intake. Therefore, to avoid any mistakes or confusion, all the high caloric food items should be removed from sight. Stuff your refrigerator only with the food that is appropriate for the sirtfood diet, and keep the juices, fruits, and vegetables ready to use. Instead of planning your meal every other day, make plans for the entire week according to the caloric limitations.

Top 20 Sirtfoods

In alphabetical order:

1. Arugula (Rocket)

2. Buckwheat

3. Capers

4. Celery

5. Chilis

6. Cocoa

7. Coffee

8. Extra Virgin Olive Oil

9. Garlic

10. Green Tea (especially Matcha)

11. Kale

12. Medjool Dates

13. Parsley

14. Red Endive

15. Red Onions

16. Red Wine

17. Soy

18. Strawberries

19. Turmeric

20. Walnuts

Additional Sirtuin Rich Foods:

Fruits

· Apples

· Blackberries

· Black currants

· Blueberries

· Citrus fruits

· Cranberries

· Goji berries

· Plums

· Raspberries

· Red Grapes

Vegetables and Herbs

· Artichokes

· Asparagus

· Broccoli

· Chia seeds

· Dill

· Green beans

· Lovage

· Quinoa

· Shallots

· Spinach

· Watercress

There are plenty of other vitamins rich and nutrient-dense plants for you to add to your meals as well. Whenever you're in doubt or looking to experiment with new ingredients, look for the freshest, seasonal produce, you can find, preferably in a wide array of colors. This combination will give you plenty of nutrition, whether or not the individual items made the top 20 list of Sirtfoods.

As you're trying out the recipes on the following pages, don't be afraid to add or swap ingredients, especially if you know you detest specific options and can't get enough of others.

This cookbook is meant to last you a lifetime, so mark up the pages and add your flair as you test out new dishes and become more and more addicted to the health and vitality of eating a diverse, nutritional diet.

Chapter 6: Phases of Sirt Food Diet

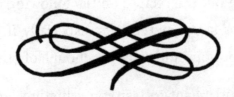

The SirtFood diet consists of two phases. I have to warn you, the first week of food is the hardest part. And you need to focus on the end of the first week, especially the early three days. Don't worry; the long-term plan is easy to follow and maintain.

The First Step:

This level is divided into two levels (days 1, 2, and 3 / days 4, 5, 6, and 7).

For days 1, 2, and 3, dieters should consume two green juices per day (including green tea, parsley, lemon, celery, arugula, and kale) and only one meal. You should limit your intake to just 1,000 calories a day.

I call this the detox/quick/juice phase, and it is generally intended for those who want to accelerate weight loss. The key, of course, is that every juice or meal contains SirtFood ingredients.

To cope with the first three days, keep an eye on the goal: lighter weight and a healthier body. And don't worry; the green juice is not that bad (I like these green juices). They also have a sumptuous dinner and can even make dark chocolates to appease your treats.

The second phase:

Congratulations! You have completed the first week of "Hardcore." The second phase is the simplest and consists of including sirtuin-based foods in your diet or daily meals. You can call this the "maintenance phase."

In this way, your body goes through the stage of burning fat and building muscle, strengthening your immune system and your general health.

In this phase, you can eat three balanced meals with SirtFood plus one green juice per day.

There is no "diet," but the choice of healthier alternatives by adding SirtFood to each meal as often as possible.

I will provide delicious cooking recipes with SirtFood to give you an idea of the excitement and health of this diet trip.

So, what happens in Phase 2 of the Sirtfood Diet?

You may repeat the two phases as often as you would like to meet your weight loss goals. Even if you have achieved it, the creators of the diet suggest adopting sirt foods for day-to-day needs because they have designed this diet as an alternative way of living.

This means that after the first three weeks, you are encouraged to keep having meals and green juices rich in sirtfoods. Other than this, here are some more things that you can do to get more and continue reaping the benefits of sirtfoods for your health:

Resume your workout routines.

Since your calorie limit for the first couple of weeks into the diet, it is best to lessen or stop working out while your body gets used to its new condition. No two persons are exactly alike, so the best thing you can do is know when you can start exercising like you usually do by paying closer attention to your body.

Most followers opt to resume their regular workout schedule after clearing phase 2 of the diet to be on the safer side. By then, you would feel more energized and more capable of completing your usual exercise sets.

Take note that even though a sirtfood diet does not require you to exercise to unlock its benefits, it would still be best for the overall wellness of your body and mind to remain fit and active every day.

Try out sirtfood smoothies with protein powder.

If you decide to start exercising again, you should add smoothies that contain lots of sirtfoods and protein powder to help you reduce the soreness of your muscles and keep you well energized throughout and after your workout.

Recipes for fun and tasty sirtfood smoothies can be found in blogs and recipe books dedicated to the Sirtfood Diet. If you are pretty confident with your skills in the kitchen, then feel free to experiment with the recommended ingredients, and discover the perfect smoothie combinations for your taste buds.

Invite your family and friends to try out the diet.

One of the best ways to maintain your healthier diet is by getting the people around you involved in it. Studies show that the kind of company you keep can have a huge influence on your lifestyle, including what and how you eat.

Ideally, you can convince them by showing the positive effects that the Sirtfood Diet has had on you. Let them read this guide so that they will have a better idea of what it is, what it can do for them, and how they should go about it.

Consider adopting the principles of the Sirtfood Diet as part of your way of life. It is just not a one-time, quick-fix meal plan, and you cannot go wrong by adding more sirtfoods into your day-to-day diet.

Chapter 7: Phase One Recipe Guide

Monday: three green juices

Breakfast: water + tea or espresso + a cup of green juice;

Lunch: green juice

Snack: a square of dark chocolate;

Dinner: Sirt meal

After dinner: a square of dark chocolate.

Drink the juices at three different times of the day (for instance, in the morning as soon as you wake, mid-morning and mid-afternoon) and choose the usual or vegan dish: pan-fried oriental prawns with buckwheat spaghetti or Miso and tofu with sesame glaze and sautéed vegetables (vegan recipe)

Tuesday: 3 green juices

Breakfast: water + tea or espresso + a cup of green juice

Lunch: 2 green juices before dinner;

Snack: a square of dark chocolate;

Dinner: Sirt meal

After dinner: a square of dark chocolate.

Welcome to Sirtfood Diet day 2. The formula is similar to that of the first day, and only the substantial meal varies. You'll have dark chocolate today, too, and the same will be valid for tomorrow. This food is so amazing we don't need an excuse to eat it.

Chocolate must be at least 85% cocoa to receive the title of a "Sirt chocolate." And even with that percentage of the various types of chocolate, not all are the same. This substance is also treated with an alkalizing agent (the so-called "Netherlands process") to reduce its acidity and give it a darker color. Unfortunately, this process dramatically reduces the activation of sirtuins by flavonoids, compromising their health benefits. Lindt Excellence 85% chocolate, is not subject to the process in the Netherlands and is therefore often recommended.

The menu includes capers on day 2, as well. Despite what many may think, they are not fruits, but buds that grow in Mediterranean countries and are picked by hand. They are high Sirt foods because they are very nutrient-rich

And quercetin and kaempferol. From the flavor standpoint, they are tiny taste concentrates. If you have never used them, feel no intimidation. You will see, if combined with the right ingredients, they will taste amazing and will give your dishes an unmistakable and inimitable aroma.

You must consume on the second day: 3 green Sirt juices and one healthy (normal or vegan) meal.

Drink the juices at three distinct times of the day (for example, when you wake up in the morning, mid-morning and mid-afternoon) and pick either the usual or vegan dish: turkey with capers, parsley and sage on spicy couscous or curly couscous cauliflower and buckwheat red onion Dahl (vegan recipe)

Wednesday: 3 green juices

Breakfast: water + tea or espresso + a cup of green juice

Lunch: 2 green juices before dinner;

Snack: a square of dark chocolate;

Dinner: Sirt meal

After dinner: a square of dark chocolate.

You are now on the third day, and even though the style is again similar to that of days 1 and 2, then the time has come to spice it with an essential ingredient. Chili has been a fundamental element of the extensive gastronomic experiences for thousands of years.

As for the health effects, we've already seen that its spiciness is perfect for activating sirtuins and stimulating metabolism. Chili's applications are endless and thus provide a simple way to eat a daily Sirt meal.

This is the last day you consume three green juices a day; you switch to two tomorrow. And we take this opportunity to browse other beverages you may have during your diet.

You will ingest three green Sirt juices and one substantial meal on the third day (regular or vegan, see below).

Drink the juices at three different times of the day (e.g., in the morning as soon as you wake up, mid-morning and mid-afternoon) and pick the usual or vegan dish: aromatic chicken breast with kale, red onion, tomato sauce, and chili or baked tofu with harissa on spicy couscous (vegan platter)

Thursday: 2 green juices

Breakfast: water + tea or espresso + a cup of green juice;

Lunch: Sirt food;

Snack: 1 green extract before dinner

Dinner: Sirt food

The Sirtfood Diet's fourth day has arrived, and you are halfway through your journey into a leaner, healthier body. The significant change from the last three days is you're only going to drink two juices instead of three, and you're going to have two solid meals in place of one. That means you'll have two green juices and two healthy snacks on the fourth day and last day, all delicious and creamy in Sirt foods. Sugar does not have any stimulating properties against sirtuins. On the contrary, it has well-known linkages with obesity, heart disease, and diabetes; in short, we target only at the antipodes of the targets. These dates, consumed in moderation, do not increase blood glucose levels as opposed to regular sugar.

You must intake on the fourth day: 2 green Sirt juices, two substantial meals (typical or vegan)

Drink the juices at various times of the day (for example the first in the morning as soon as you wake up or in the middle of the morning, the second in the middle of the afternoon) and select the regular or vegan dishes: muesli sirt, pan-fried salmon filet with caramelized chicory, rocket salad and celery leaves or muesli Sirt and Tuscan stewed beans (vegan recipe)

Friday: 2 green juices

Breakfast: water + tea or espresso + a cup of green juice

Lunch: Sirt food

Snack: a green extract before dinner;

Dinner: Sirt food

You have hit the fifth day, so it's time to add some berries. Because of its high sugar content, the fruit was the subject of the lousy advertisement. That is not applicable to berries. The sugar content of strawberries is shallow: one teaspoon per 100 grams. They also have a significant influence on how simple sugars are processed in the body.

Scientists have found that this causes a reduction in insulin demand if we add strawberries to simple sugars, and thus transforms food into a machine that releases energy for a long time to come. Therefore fruits are a perfect diet element that will help you lose weight and get back into shape. They are also delicious and extremely versatile, as you'll discover the fresh and light Middle Eastern tabbouleh in the Sirt version.

The Miso is a famous Japanese soup made from fermented soy. Miso has an overpowering scent of umami, a complete explosion for the taste buds. We know better the monosodium glutamate in our modern society, produced artificially to replicate the same feeling. Needless to say, deriving the magical umami taste from conventional and natural ingredients, full of beneficial substances, is much more preferable. It is found in all good supermarkets and healthy food stores in the form of a paste and should be present in each kitchen to give many different dishes a touch of taste.

Because umami flavors enhance one another, Miso is correctly associated with other tasty / umami foods, particularly when it comes to cooked proteins, as you will discover in the delicious, quick, and easy dishes you are going to eat today.

You will ingest two green Sirt juices and two solid (regular or vegan) meals on the fifth day.

Drink the juices at various times of the day (for instance; the first in the middle of the morning or as soon as you wake up; the second in the middle of the afternoon) and pick the usual or vegan dishes: buckwheat Tabbouleh with strawberries, baked cod marinated in Miso with sautéed.

Sesame or buckwheat vegetables and strawberry Tabbouleh (vegan platter) and kale (vegan dish).

Saturday: 2 green juices

Breakfast: water + tea or espresso + a cup of green juice

Lunch: Sirt food

Snack: a green extract before dinner;

Dinner: Sirt food

There is no better Sirt food than olive oil and red wine. Virgin olive oil is only obtained by mechanical means from the fruit, in conditions that do not deteriorate it, so you can be sure of its quality and polyphenol content. "Extra virgin" oil is the first pressing oil ("virgin" is the product of the second pressing) and thus has more flavor and higher quality: this is what we highly prefer to use while cooking.

No Sirt menu would be complete without red wine, which is one of the diet's cornerstones. It contains resveratrol and piceatannol sirtuins activators that are likely to explain the longevity and slenderness associated with the traditional French way of life and that are at the root of the enthusiasm unleashed by Sirt foods.

You'll expect two green Sirt juices and two strong (regular or vegan) meals on the sixth day.

Drink the juices at different times of the day (for example, the first in the middle of the morning or as soon as you wake up, the second in the middle of the afternoon) and choose the ordinary or vegan dishes: Super Sirt salad and grilled beef fillet with red wine sauce, onion rings, curly garlic kale and roasted potatoes with aromatic herbs, or

Super lentil Sirt salad (vegan dish) and red bean mole sauce with roasted potato (vegan recipe).

Sunday: 2 green juices

Breakfast: a bowl of Sirt Muesli + a cup of green juice

Lunch: Sirt food

Snack: a cup of green juice;

Dinner: Sirt food

The seventh day is the final of the diet's step 1. Instead of seeing it as an end, see it as a beginning, for you are about to embark on a new life in which sirt foods can play a central role in your diet. Today's menu is a perfect example of how easy it is to integrate them into your daily diet in abundance. Just take your favorite dishes, and turn them into a Sirt banquet with a pinch of imagination.

Walnuts are perfect Sirt food because they refute current views. They have high-fat content and many calories, yet they have shown to contribute to weight reduction and metabolic diseases, all thanks to sirtuin activation. Also, they are a versatile ingredient, excellent in baked dishes, salads, and alone as a snack.

We can apply the same reasoning to a dish that is easy to prepare, such as an omelet. The plate must be the traditional recipe that the whole family appreciates, and it must be easy to turn into a Sirt dish with a few little tricks. We use bacon in our recycling. Why? For what? Just because it just fits perfectly. The Sirtfood Diet tells us what to include, not what to exclude, which allows us to change our eating habits in the long term. Isn't that, after all, the secret of not getting the lost pounds back and staying healthy?

You'll assume two green Sirt juices on the seventh day; 2 solid (typical or vegan) meals.

Drink the juices at different times of the day (for example the first in the morning as soon as you wake up or in the middle of the morning, the second in the middle of the afternoon). Choose the traditional or vegan dishes: omelet sirt and boiled aubergine wedges with walnut and parsley pesto and tomato salad (vegan recipe).

There are no calorie restrictions during the second phase but indications on which Sirt foods should be eaten to consolidate weight loss and not run the risk of getting the kilograms lost back.

Chapter 8: Phase Two Recipe Guide

Phase 2: Maintenance

Congratulations,

You have finished the first "hardcore" week. The second step is the

simpler one and is the actual integration of food choices loaded with sirtuin

into your daily diet or meals. You can call this the "stage of maintenance."

Your body will be subjected to the fat-burning level, and muscle gain plus a boost to your immune system and overall health.

You can now get three healthy SirtFood-filled meals per day for this process plus one green juice per day. There is no "dieting" but more about selecting safer alternatives with as much as possible, adding SirtFood to every meal. I will be providing some SirtFood inclusive recipes for tasty dishes to give you an idea of how exciting and healthy this diet journey is. Now you are going back to a daily intake of calories intending to keep your weight loss stable and your Sirtfood intake high. You should have undergone a degree of weight loss by now, but you should still feel trimming and revitalizing. Phase 2 lasts for 14 days. During this time you will eat three sirtfood-rich meals, one sirtfood-green juice and up to 2 free snacks of Sirtfood bite. Strict calorie-counting is actively discouraged if you follow recommendations and eat reasonable portions of balanced meals; you shouldn't feel hungry or consume too much. You will have the same drinks you drank in step 1. With the small improvement, you're welcome to enjoy the occasional glass of red wine (though you don't drink more than three a week).

How to Follow Phase 2

The key to success in this process is having your diet packed full of Sirtfoods. We've put together a seven-day meal schedule to adapt to make it as easy as possible, with tasty family-friendly meals, filled with Sirtfoods every day to the rafters. Now what you need to do is to implement the seven-day program twice to fulfill Phase 2's fourteen days. On each of fourteen days, your diet will consist of: Three times balanced sirtfood meals 1-time sirtfood green juice 1 – 2 times free sirtfood snacks Also when you have to eat those; there are no strict laws. Be agile throughout every day and suit them. Two basic thumb-rules are: Take sirtfood green juice either in the morning or at least half an hour before breakfast. Try your best to make dinner by 7 PM.

Portion Sizes

In Phase 2, our attention is not on calorie counting. For the average person, this is not a practical approach or a good one over the long term. Instead, we concentrate on healthy servings, really well-balanced meals, and most notably, filling up on Sirt

Foods so that you can continue to benefit from their fat-burning and health-promoting impact. We've even designed the meals in the plan to make them satiate, making you stay full for longer. This, coupled with Sirtfoods' innate appetite-regulating power, ensures you're not going to spend 14 days feeling thirsty, but rather comfortably fulfilled, well-fed, and highly well-nourished. Just like in Phase 1, try to listen and be driven by your appetite. When you prepare meals according to our guidelines and notice that you are comfortably full before you finish a meal, then stop eating is perfectly fine!

What to Drink

During Phase 2 you'll need to include one green juice every day. This is to keep you top with high Sirt Foods prices. Just like in Phase 1, you will quickly absorb other fluids in Phase 2. Our preferred

beverages contain remaining plain water, bottled flavored water, coffee, and green tea. Whether black or white tea is your preference, feel free to enjoy it. The same goes for herbal teas. The best news is that during Phase 2, you will enjoy the occasional bottle of red wine. Due to its content of sirtuin-activating polyphenols, particularly resveratrol and piceatannol, red wine is a sirtfood that makes it the best choice of alcoholic beverage. However, with alcohol itself causing adverse effects on our fat cells, restraint is still safest, so we suggest restricting the drink to one glass of red wine with a meal for two to three days a week in Phase 2.

Returning Three Meals

You enjoyed only one or two meals per day during Phase 1 and allowed you plenty of versatility when you eat your meals. As we are now back to a more normal routine and the well-tested practice of three meals a day, learning about breakfast is a good time. We are eating a good breakfast that sets us on for the day, raising our levels of energy and focus. Eating early holds our blood sugar and fat rates in balance, in terms of our metabolism. Several studies point out that breakfast is a good thing, usually showing that people who eat breakfast are less prone to become overweight. The explanation for this is because of our internal clocks inside. Our bodies ask us to feed early in expectation of when we will be busiest and need food. Yet, as many as a third of us will miss breakfasts on any given day. It's a classic symptom in our crazy modern life, and the feeling is there's simply not enough time to eat correctly. But as you will see, with the nifty breakfasts we have laid out for you, nothing could be further from the truth. Whether it's the Sirtfood smoothie that can be drunk on the go, the premade Sirt muesli, or the quick and easy Sirtfood scrambled eggs/tofu, finding those extra few minutes in the morning will reap dividends not only for your day but for your longer-term weight and health. With Sirtfoods functioning to overcharge our energy levels, there's, even more, to learn from getting a hit from them early in the morning to continue your day. This is done not only by consuming a Sirtfood-rich meal but also by including the green juice, which we suggest you have either first thing in the morning — at least thirty minutes before breakfast— or mid-morning. We get a lot of reports from our personal experience of people who first consume their green juice and don't feel hungry for a few hours afterward. If this is the impact it's having on you, taking a couple of hours until having breakfast is perfectly fine. Just don't miss this one. Instead of a good breakfast, you should kick off your day and then wait two to three hours to have the green juice. Be versatile, and just go with anything that suits you.

Bi-weekly menu

In addition to our standard plan, we also have a meatless version that is suitable for vegetarians and vegans. You can also mix it with anything you want. You will consume every day. Three balanced Sirtfood meals One green juice sirt food 1 to 2 optional sirt food snacks

At this point, you can eat any sort-based meal as long as you have one sirt food juice per day.

This contains recipes to help you stay in the maintenance phase, phase 2. The other great advantage of these phase 2 recipes is that you cannot use them only in the maintenance phase to maintain the loss of weights and changes. That you worked so hard to see. You can use it forever.

Again, you can duplicate and keep some of the recipes. However, don't forget to eat them as soon as possible to get all these valuable and perishable antioxidant properties!

Breakfast

- Green Omelette
- 234 calories
- Served 1 • Ready in 10 minutes
- 2 large eggs at room temperature
- 1 shallot, peeled and chopped
- Handful of arugula
- 3 sprigs of chopped parsley
- 1 teaspoon extra virgin olive oil
- Salt and black pepper

Beat the eggs in a small bowl and set aside—Fry the shallot for 5 minutes over medium heat with a little oil. Pour the eggs into the saucepans and stir the mixture for a second.

Turn the eggs over medium heat and brown them just enough so that the loose eggs run on the burner for less than a minute. Add vegetables, herbs, and spices as it is still sweet. TIP: You don't even have to turn it over, as you can also simmer the egg (be careful not to burn it).

TIP: Another option is to put it in a roasting oven for 3 to 5 minutes (check if it is until it is golden but burnt).

Oatmeal for cobbler's breakfasts

- 241 calories
- For 2 people
- 2 cups ready-to-eat oats / uncooked flakes

- 1 cup blackcurrant without stalks
- 1 teaspoon of honey (or ¼ teaspoon of raw sugar)
- ½ cup of water (try more or less to try the pan)
- 1 cup plain yogurt (or soy or coconut)

Boil the berries, honey, and water, then simmer. Place in a glass container in the refrigerator until it is fresh and ready (about 30 minutes or more).

When you're ready to eat, place the berries on the oatmeal and yogurt. Serve immediately.

Apple and blackcurrant pancakes

- 337 calories
- For 4 people
- 2 apples, cut into small pieces
- Quickly cook 2 cups rolled oats
- 1 cup of flour of your choice
- 1 teaspoon of baking soda
- 2 Tablespoons of raw sugar, coconut sugar, or 2 tablespoons. Hot and easy to spread honey
- 2 egg whites
- 1 ¼ cup milk (or soy / rice / coconut)
- 2 A teaspoon of extra virgin olive oil
- a pinch of salt

For the berry garnish:

- 1 cup blackcurrant, washed and stemmed less
- 3 tablespoons of water (you can use less)
- 2 tablespoons of sugar (see above for types)

Place the garnish ingredients on low heat in a saucepan and frequently stir for about 10 minutes until cooked and the juices are released.

Take the dry ingredients and mix them in a bowl. Then add the apples and process them one by one (you can't use everything) until they are well chopped. Beat the egg whites well and mix gently in the pancake batter. Set aside in the refrigerator.

Pour a quarter of the oil into a flat pan or frying pan and, when hot, pour the batter into a pancake. If the pancakes have golden edges and form air bubbles, they can be easily turned over.

Test if the bottom can move away from the pan before turning it over. Repeat for the three pancakes. Cover each pancake with berries.

Muesli - The Art Form

Served 1st

Ingredients:

- 1 cup buckwheat puffs
- 1 cup buckwheat flakes (ready to eat, but not whole wheat to cook) ½ cup coconut flakes
- ½ cup Medjool dates, cored, cut into smaller and smaller pieces

- 1 cup cocoa beans or very dark chocolate chips
- 1/2 cup chopped nuts
- One cup chopped stemless strawberries 1 cup Greek yogurt or coconut or soy.

Manual:

Mix without garnish with yogurt and strawberries.

You can store up to a week. Keep in a tightly closed case. Add toppings (even different berries or different yogurts.

You can even use berry toppings while learning how to do it with other recipes.

Chapter 9: 7 Day Meal Plan

Days	Breakfast	Main	Dinner
1	Pancakes with Apples and Blackcurrants	Butternut pumpkin with buckwheat	Tofu Thai Curry
2	Black Forest Smoothie	Pasta with kale and black olive	Beans & Kale Soup
3	Buckwheat Pancakes	Butter Bean and Miso Dip with Celery Sticks and Oatcakes	Lentils & Greens Soup
4	Vegetable & Nut Loaf	Spiced Scrambled Eggs	Asian Slaw
5	Buckwheat Porridge	Shitake soup with tofu	Egg Fried Buckwheat
6	Chocolate Waffles	Chicken curry with potatoes and kale	Aromatic Ginger Turmeric Buckwheat
7	Miso and Sesame-Glazed Tofu with Chili Stir-Fried Greens and Ginger	Buckwheat noodles with salmon and rocket	Kale and Corn Succotash

Notwithstanding our standard arrangement, we additionally have a sans meat variant, which is appropriate for the two veggie lovers and vegetarians. Don't hesitate to go with whichever one you like, or even blend and match.

Every day you will consume: 1 x Sirtfood green juice.

Chapter 10: Breakfast

Day 1 - Pancakes with Apples and Blackcurrants

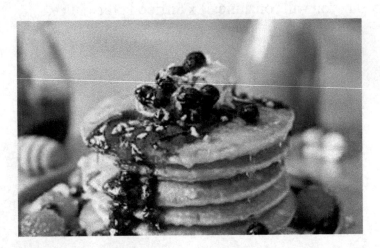

Preparation time: 30 min

Cooking time: 10 min

Servings: 4

Ingredients:

2 Apples, cut into small chunks

2 cups of quick-cooking oats

1 cup flour of your choice

1 Tsp. baking powder

2 tbsp. raw sugar, coconut sugar, or 2 tbsp. honey that is warm and easy to distribute

2 egg whites

1 ¼ cups of milk (or soy/rice/coconut)

2 tsp. extra virgin olive oil

A dash of salt

For the berry topping:

1 cup blackcurrants, washed and stalks removed

3 tbsp. water (may use less)

2 tbsp. sugar (see above for types)

Directions:

Place the ingredients for the topping in a small pot simmer, frequently stirring for about 10 minutes until it cooks down and releases the juices.

Take the dry ingredients and mix them in a bowl. After, add the apples and the milk a bit at a time (you may not use it all), until it is a batter. Stiffly whisk the egg whites and then gently mix them into the pancake batter. Set aside in the refrigerator.

Pour a one-quarter of the oil onto a flat pan or flat griddle. When hot, pour some of the batters into it in a pancake shape. When the pancakes start to have golden brown edges and form air bubbles, they may be ready to be gently flipped.

Test to be sure the bottom can change life away from the pan before actually flipping. Repeat for the three pancakes. Top each pancake with the berries.

Nutrition: 337 calories

Day 2 - Black Forest Smoothie

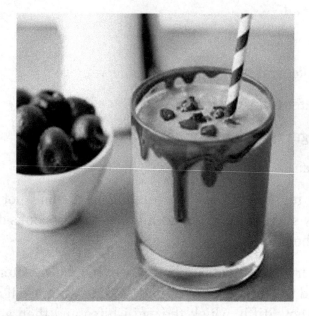

Preparation Time: 10 Minutes

Cooking time: 0 Minutes

Servings: 2

Ingredients

100g (3½oz) frozen cherries

25g (1oz) kale

1 Medjool date

1 tablespoon cocoa powder

2 teaspoons chia seeds

200mls (7fl oz) milk or soya milk

Directions:

Place all the ingredients into a blender and process until smooth and creamy.

Nutrition:

Calories: 232 Calories

Total Fat: 4g

Saturated Fat: 1g

Sodium: 229mg

Carbohydrates: 53g

Fiber: 10g

Sugar: 29g

Protein: 5g

Day 3 - Buckwheat Pancakes

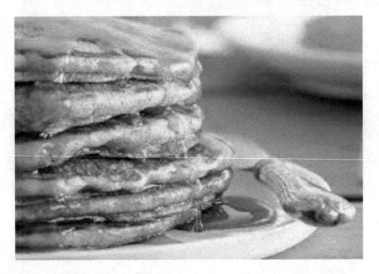

Preparation Time: 15 minutes

Cooking Time: 15 minutes

Servings: 5

Ingredients:

1 cup of coconut milk

2 teaspoons apple cider vinegar

1 cup buckwheat flour

2 tablespoons ground flax seed

1 tablespoon baking powder

¼ teaspoon of sea salt

¼ cup maple syrup

1 teaspoon vanilla extract

1 tablespoon coconut oil

Directions:

In a medium bowl, mix the coconut milk and vinegar. Set aside.

In a large bowl, mix the flour, flaxseed, baking powder, and salt.

Add the coconut milk mixture, maple syrup, and vanilla extract and beat until well combined.

In a nonstick skillet, melt coconut oil over medium heat.

Place about 1/3 cup of the mixture and spread in an even circle.

Cook for about 1-2 minutes.

Flip and cook for an additional 1 minute then remove from the pan.

Repeat with the remaining mixture.

Serve warm.

Nutrition

Calories 143.

Total fat 3 g.

Saturated fat Trace.

Trans fat 0 g.

Monounsaturated fat 2 g.

Cholesterol Trace.

Day 4 - Vegetable & Nut Loaf

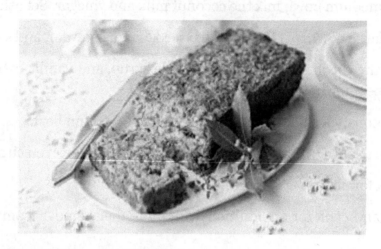

Preparation Time: 10 Minutes

Cooking time: 30 Minutes

Servings: 3

Ingredients

175g (6oz) mushrooms, finely chopped

100g (3½ oz) haricot beans

100g (3½ oz) walnuts, finely chopped

100g (3½ oz) peanuts, finely chopped

1 carrot, finely chopped

3 sticks celery, finely chopped

1 bird's-eye chili, finely chopped

1 red onion, finely chopped

1 egg, beaten

2 cloves of garlic, chopped

2 tablespoons olive oil

2 teaspoons turmeric powder

2 tablespoons soy sauce

4 tablespoons fresh parsley, chopped

100mls (3½ fl oz) water

60mls (2fl oz) red wine

Directions

Heat the oil in a pan and add the garlic, chili, carrot, celery, onion, mushrooms and turmeric. Cook for 5 minutes. Place the haricot beans in a bowl and stir in nuts, vegetables, soy sauce, egg, parsley, red wine, and water. Grease and line a large loaf tin with greaseproof paper. Spoon the mixture into the loaf tin, cover it with foil, and bake in the oven at 190C/375F for 60-90 minutes. Let it stand for 10 minutes then turn onto a serving plate.

Nutrition

Calories 297.3.

Total fat 17.9 g.

Saturated fat Trace 3.0 g.

Trans fat 0 g.

Monounsaturated fat 7.3 g.

Cholesterol Trace 98.3 mg.

Day 5 - Buckwheat Porridge

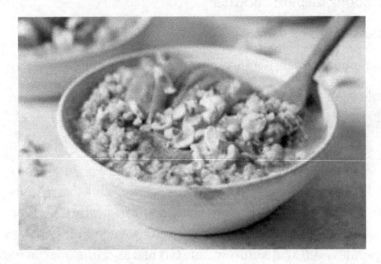

Preparation Time: 10 minutes

Cooking Time: 15 minutes

Servings: 2

Ingredients:

1 cup buckwheat, rinsed

1 cup unsweetened almond milk

1 cup of water

½ teaspoon ground cinnamon

½ teaspoon vanilla extract

1-2 tablespoons raw honey

¼ cup fresh blueberries

Directions:

In a nonstick saucepan, add all ingredients except honey and blueberries over medium-high heat and bring it to a boil.

78

Now, reduce the heat to low and simmer, covered for about 10 minutes.

Stir in the honey and remove the pan of porridge from heat.

Set aside, covered, for about 5 minutes.

With a fork, fluff the mixture and transfer into serving bowls.

Top with blueberries and serve.

Nutrition

5.68 g of protein.

1.04 g of fat.

33.5 g of carbohydrate.

4.5 g of fiber.

148 milligrams (mg) of potassium.

118 mg of phosphorus.

86 mg of magnesium.

12 mg of calcium.

Day 6 -Chocolate Waffles

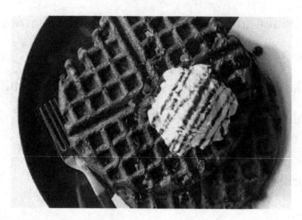

Preparation Time: 15 minutes

Cooking Time: 24 minutes

Servings: 8

Ingredients:

2 cups unsweetened almond milk

1 tablespoon fresh lemon juice

1 cup buckwheat flour

½ cup cacao powder

¼ cup flaxseed meal

1 teaspoon baking soda

1 teaspoon baking powder

¼ teaspoons kosher salt

2 large eggs

½ cup coconut oil, melted

¼ cup dark brown sugar

2 teaspoons vanilla extract

2 ounces unsweetened dark chocolate, chopped roughly

Directions:

In a bowl, add the almond milk and lemon juice and mix well.

Set aside for about 10 minutes.

Place buckwheat flour, cacao powder, flaxseed meal, baking soda, baking powder, and salt and mix well in a bowl.

In the bowl of the almond milk mixture, place the eggs, coconut oil, brown sugar, and vanilla extract and beat until smooth.

Now, place the flour mixture and beat until smooth.

Gently fold in the chocolate pieces.

Preheat the waffle iron and then grease it.

Place the desired amount of the mixture into the preheated waffle iron and cook for about 3 minutes or until golden brown.

Repeat with the remaining mixture.

Serve warm.

Nutrition:

Calories 297.3.

Total fat 10.1 g.

Saturated fat Trace 3.57 g.

Trans fat 0 g.

Monounsaturated fat 2.56 g.

Cholesterol Trace 98.3 mg.

Day 7 - Miso and Sesame-Glazed Tofu with Chili Stir-Fried Greens and Ginger

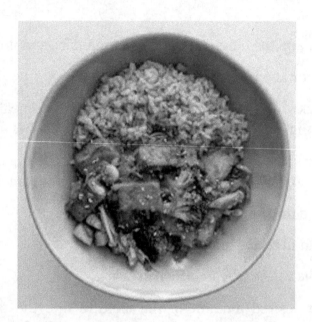

Preparation Time: 10 Minutes

Cooking time: 60 Minutes

Servings: 3

Ingredients:

1 tablespoon mirin

1 ounce miso paste

Ounces block firm tofu

 2 ounces trimmed celery (it should be ⅓ cup

After being sliced)

 ¼ cup red onion, sliced

 4–5 ounces (1 small) zucchini (it should be 1

cup when sliced)

1 Thai chili

2 garlic cloves

1 teaspoon fresh ginger, finely chopped

2 ounces (¾ cup) kale, chopped

2 teaspoons sesame seeds

1 ounce (¼ cup) buckwheat

1 teaspoon ground turmeric

2 teaspoons extra-virgin olive oil

1 teaspoon tamari (or soy sauce for

gluten-free meals)

Directions:

Preheat the oven at 400 degrees Fahrenheit.

On a small roasting pan, line some parchment paper.

Mix the miso and mirin.

Then you will need to cut the tofu lengthways. Each

piece has to be cut diagonally in half to get triangles.

You will need to cover the tofu with miso mixture. Let it

marinate while you prepare the rest.

Cut the red onion, celery, and zucchini on the angle, and

then chop the ginger, garlic, and chili. Put them aside.

Then you will have to cook the kale in a steamer for 5

minutes. Remove it and put it aside.

Then, you will need to place the tofu in the roasting

pan. Sprinkle sesame seeds on it, and let it roast in the oven for 15 to 20 minutes until you see it nicely caramelized.

After it is cooked, you will need to drain them.

Take a frying pan and place it over high heat.

Pour the oil in it, then add zucchini, celery, onion,

ginger, chili, and garlic. Let them fry for 1 to 2 minutes.

Lower the heat to medium, and let it cook for 3 to 4

minutes until you see the veggies cooked and still crunchy.

It is not a bad idea to add 1 tablespoon of water if you

notice the vegetables sticking to the pan.

Add the kale and tamari sauce (for a final touch) and

cook it for one minute.

When you have the tofu ready, serve it with buckwheat and

greens.

NUTRITION:

- Calories per serving 164
- Fat per serving 10.1g
- Saturated fat per serving 1.4g
- Monounsaturated fat per serving 3.5g
- Polyunsaturated fat per serving 5.2g
- Protein per serving 12g
- Carbohydrate per serving 8g
- Fiber per serving 3g
- Cholesterol per serving 0.0mg
- Iron per serving 2mg
- Sodium per serving 152mg
- Calcium per serving 78mg

Chapter 11: Lunch

Day 1 - Butternut pumpkin with buckwheat

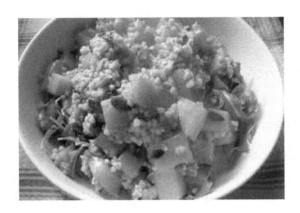

Preparation Time: 5 Minutes

Cooking time: 50 Minutes

Servings: 4

Ingredients

One tablespoon of extra virgin olive oil

One red onion, finely chopped

One tablespoon fresh ginger, finely chopped

Three cloves of garlic, finely chopped

Two small chilies, finely chopped

One tablespoon cumin

One cinnamon stick

Two tablespoons turmeric

800g chopped canned tomatoes

300ml vegetable broth

100g dates, seeded and chopped

one 400g tin of chickpeas, drained

500g butter squash, peeled, seeded and cut into pieces

200g buckwheat

5g coriander, chopped

10g parsley, chopped

Directions

Preheat the oven to 400 °.

Heat the olive oil in a frying pan and sauté the onion, ginger, garlic, and Thai chili. After two minutes, add cumin, cinnamon, and turmeric and cook for another two minutes while stirring.

Add the tomatoes, dates, stock, and chickpeas, stir well and cook over low heat for 45 to 60 minutes. Add some water as required. In the meantime, mix the pumpkin pieces with olive oil. Bake in the oven for about 30 minutes until soft.

Cook the buckwheat according to the Directions and add the remaining turmeric. When everything is cooked, add the pumpkin to the other ingredients in the roaster and serve with the buckwheat. Sprinkle with coriander and parsley.

Nutrition:

Calories per serving 248.1

Total Fat .8.7g

Saturated fat per serving 2.6g

Monounsaturated fat per serving 1.5g

Polyunsaturated fat per serving 4.0g

Protein per serving 8.5g

Day 2 - Pasta with kale and Black Olive

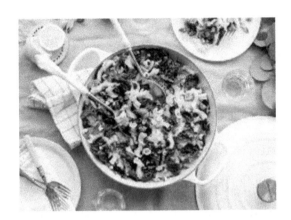

Preparation time: 10 minutes

Cooking time: 40 minutes

Servings: 3

Ingredients:

60 g of buckwheat pasta

180 gr of pasta

Six leaves of washed curly kale

20 black olives

Two tablespoons of oil

½ chili pepper

Directions:

Cut the curly kale leaves into strips about 4 cm wide; cook them in salted boiling water for 5 minutes. Also, add the pasta to the pan. While the pasta is cooking, in a non-stick pan, towards the oil and olives. Drain the pasta and cabbage (keeping some cooking water aside) and add them to the olives. Mix well, adding, if needed, a little cooking water. Add the chili pepper and keep everything well.

Nutrition:

Calories per serving 372.7 g

Total Fat .28.0g

Saturated fat per serving 2.7g

Monounsaturated fat per serving 10.0g

Polyunsaturated fat per serving 2.1g

Protein per serving 3.6g

Day 3 - Butter Bean and Miso Dip with Celery Sticks and Oatcakes

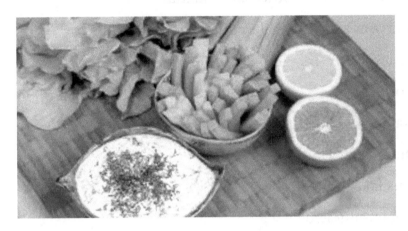

Preparation Time: 5 Minutes

Cooking time: 55 Minutes

Servings: 4

Ingredients

2 x 14-ounce cans (400g each) of butter beans, drained and rinsed

Three tablespoons extra virgin olive oil

Two tablespoons brown miso paste

Juice and grated zest of

1/2 unwaxed lemon

Four medium scallions, trimmed and finely chopped

One garlic clove, crushed

1/4 Thai chili, finely chopped celery sticks, to serve

Oatcakes, to serve

Directions

1. Simply mash the first seven ingredients together with a potato masher until you have a coarse mixture.

2. Serve as a dip with celery sticks and oatcakes.

Nutrition:

Calories 143.

Total fat 3 g.

Saturated fat Trace.

Trans fat 0 g.

Monounsaturated fat 2 g.

Cholesterol Trace.

Day 4 - Spiced Scrambled Eggs

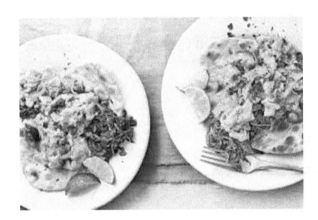

Preparation Time: 5 Minutes

Cooking time: 15 Minutes

Servings: 4

Ingredients

One teaspoon extra virgin olive oil

1/8 cup (20g) red onion, finely chopped

1/2 Thai chili, finely chopped

Three medium eggs

1/4 cup (50ml) milk

One teaspoon ground turmeric

Two tablespoons (5g) parsley, finely chopped

Directions

1. Heat the oil in a frying pan and fry the red onion and chili until soft but not browned.

2. Whisk together the eggs, milk, turmeric, and parsley.

3. Add to the hot pan and continue cooking over low to medium heat, continually moving the egg mixture around the pan to scramble it and stop it from sticking/burning.

4. When you have achieved your desired consistency, serve.

Nutrition:

Calories 218.2.

Total fat 15.3 g.

Saturated fat Trace 6.3 g.

Trans fat 0 g.

Monounsaturated fat 5.5 g.

Cholesterol Trace. 386.9 mg

Day 5 - Shitake Soup with Tofu

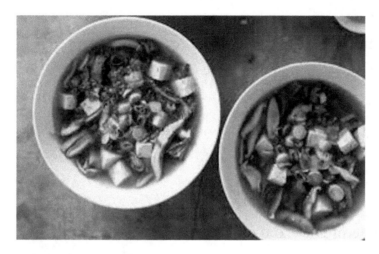

Preparation Time: 5 Minutes

Cooking time: 15 Minutes

Servings: 4

Ingredients

10g dried Wakame algae (instant)

1-liter vegetable stock

200g shitake mushrooms, sliced

120g miso paste

400g natural tofu, cut into cubes

Two spring onions

One red chili, chopped

Directions

Bring the stock to boil, add the mushrooms, and cook for 2 minutes. In the meantime, dissolve the miso paste in a bowl with some warm stock, put it back into the pot together with the tofu, do not let it boil anymore. Soak the Wakame as needed (on the packet), add the spring onions and Tai Chi, and stir again and serve.

Nutrition:

Calories 137.4.

Total fat 6.7 g.

Saturated fat Trace 1.0 g.

Trans fat 0 g.

Monounsaturated fat 1.8 g.

Cholesterol Trace. 0.0 mg

Day 6 - Chicken Curry with Potatoes And Kale

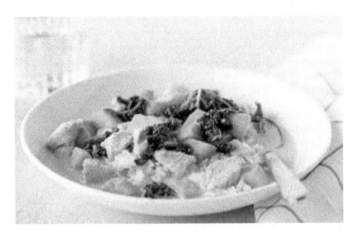

Preparation Time: 5 Minutes

Cooking time: 45 Minutes

Servings: 4

Ingredients

600g chicken breast, cut into pieces

Four tablespoons of extra virgin olive oil

Three tablespoons turmeric

Two red onions, sliced

Two red chilies, finely chopped

Three cloves of garlic, finely chopped

One tablespoon freshly chopped ginger

One tablespoon curry powder

One tin of small tomatoes (400ml)

500ml chicken broth

200ml coconut milk

Two pieces cardamom

One cinnamon stick

600g potatoes (mainly waxy)

10g parsley, chopped

175g kale, chopped

5g coriander, chopped

Directions

Marinate the chicken in a teaspoon of olive oil and a tablespoon of turmeric for about 30 minutes. Then fry in a high frying pan at high heat for about 4 minutes. Remove from the pan and set aside.

Heat a tablespoon of oil in a pan with chili, garlic, onion, and ginger. Boil everything over medium heat and then add the curry powder and a tablespoon of turmeric and cook for another two minutes, stirring occasionally. Add tomatoes, cook for another two minutes until finally chicken stock, coconut milk, cardamom, and cinnamon stick are added. Cook for about 45 to 60 minutes and add some broth if necessary.

In the meantime, preheat the oven to 425 °. Peel and chop the potatoes. Bring water to the boil, add the vegetables with turmeric, and cook for 5 minutes. Then pour off the water and let it evaporate for about 10 minutes. Spread olive oil with the potatoes on a baking tray and bake in the oven for 30 minutes.

When the potatoes and curry are almost ready, add the coriander, kale, and chicken and cook for five minutes until the chicken is hot.

Add parsley to the potatoes and serve with the chicken curry.

Nutrition:

Calories 894

Carbs 162g

Fat 22g

Protein 25g

Fiber 26g

Net carbs 136g

Sodium 2447mg

Cholesterol 0mg

Day 7 - Buckwheat Noodles with Salmon And Rocket

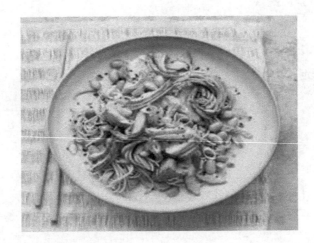

Preparation Time: 5 Minutes

Cooking time: 45 Minutes

Servings: 4

Ingredients

Two tablespoons of extra virgin olive oil

One red onion, finely chopped

Two cloves of garlic, finely chopped

Two red chilies, finely chopped

150g cherry tomatoes halved

100ml white wine

300g buckwheat noodles

250g smoked salmon

Two tablespoons of capers

Juice of half a lemon

60g rocket salad

10g parsley, chopped

Directions

Heat 1 teaspoon of the oil in a coated pan, add onions, garlic, and chili at medium temperature and fry briefly. Then add the tomatoes and the white wine to the pan and allow the wine to reduce.

Cook the pasta according to the Directions.

In the meantime, cut the salmon into strips, and when the pasta is ready, add it to the pan together with the capers, lemon juice, capers rocket, remaining olive oil, and parsley and mix Done.

Nutrition:

Calories 320.1

Carbs. 25.2

Fat 13.0 g

Protein 27.0 g

Chapter 12:Dinner

Day 1 - Tofu Thai Curry

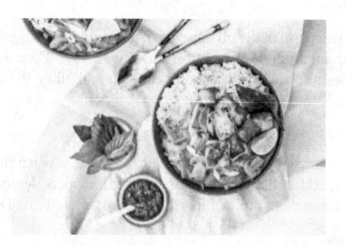

Preparation Time: 5 Minutes

Cooking time: 65 Minutes

Servings: 2

Ingredients

400g (14oz) tofu, diced

200g (7oz) sugar snaps peas

5cm (2 inches) chunk fresh ginger root, peeled and finely chopped

2 red onions, chopped

2 cloves of garlic, crushed

2 bird's eye chilies

2 tablespoons tomato puree

1 stalk of lemongrass, inner stalks only

1 tablespoon fresh coriander (cilantro), chopped

1 teaspoon cumin

300mls (½ pint) coconut milk

200mls (7fl oz) vegetable stock (broth)

1 tablespoon virgin olive oil

Juice of 1 lime

Directions

Heat the oil in a frying pan, add the onion and cook for 4 minutes. Add in the chilies, cumin, ginger, and garlic and cook for 2 minutes. Add the tomato puree, lemongrass, sugar-snap peas, lime juice, and tofu and cook for 2 minutes. Pour in the stock (broth), coconut milk and coriander (cilantro) and simmer for 5 minutes. Serve with brown rice or buckwheat and a handful of rockets (arugula) leaves on the side.

Nutrition:

Calories 346.3.

Total fat 26.4 g.

Saturated fat Trace 2.0 g.

Trans fat 0 g.

Monounsaturated fat 5.4 g.

Cholesterol Trace. 0.0 mg

Day 2 - Beans & Kale Soup

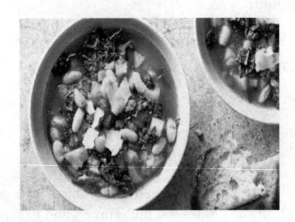

Preparation Time: 15 minutes

Cooking Time: 30 minutes

 Servings: 6

Ingredients:

2 tablespoons olive oil

2 onions, chopped

4 garlic cloves, minced

1-pound kale, tough ribs removed and chopped

2 (14-ounce) cans cannellini beans, rinsed and drained

6 cups of water

Salt and ground black pepper, as required

Directions

In a large pan, heat the oil over medium heat and sauté the onion and garlic for about 4-5 minutes.

Add the kale and cook for about 1-2 minutes.

Add beans, water, salt, and black pepper and bring to a boil.

Cook partially covered for about 15-20 minutes.

Serve hot.

Nutrition:

Calories 270.4.

Total fat 4.7 g.

Saturated fat Trace 0.6 g.

Trans fat 0 g.

Monounsaturated fat 2.6 g.

Cholesterol Trace. 0.0 mg

Day 3 - Lentils & Greens Soup

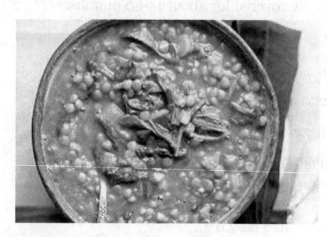

Preparation Time: 15 minutes

Cooking Time: 55 minutes

Servings: 6

Ingredients:

1 tablespoon olive oil

2 carrots, peeled and chopped

2 celery stalks, chopped

1 medium red onion, chopped

3 garlic cloves, minced

1½ teaspoon ground cumin

1 teaspoon ground turmeric

¼ teaspoon red pepper flakes

1 (14½-ounce) can diced tomatoes

1 cup red lentils, rinsed

5½ cups water

2 cups fresh mustard greens, chopped

Salt and ground black pepper, as required

2 tablespoons fresh lemon juice

Directions:

Heat olive oil in a large pan over medium heat and sauté the carrots, celery, and onion for about 5-6 minutes.

Add the garlic and spices and sauté for about 1 minute.

Add the tomatoes and cook for about 2-3 minutes.

Stir in the lentils and water and bring to a boil.

Now, reduce the heat to low and simmer, covered for about 35 minutes.

Stir in greens and cook for about 5 minutes.

Stir in salt, black pepper, and lemon juice and remove from the heat.

Serve hot.

Nutrition:

Calories 167.4

Total fat 5.5 g.

Saturated fat Trace 1.2 g.

Trans fat 0 g.

Monounsaturated fat 4.3 g.

Cholesterol Trace. 3.3 mg

Day 4 - Asian Slaw

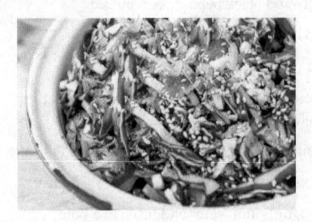

Preparation Time: 5 Minutes

Cooking time: 25 Minutes

Servings: 2

Ingredients:

Red cabbage, shredded – 2 cups

Broccoli florets, chopped – 2 cups

Carrots, shredded – 1 cup

Red onion, finely sliced – 1

Red bell pepper, finely sliced - .5

Cilantro, chopped - .5 cup

Sesame seeds – 1 tablespoon

Peanuts, chopped - .5 cup

Sriracha – 2 teaspoons

Rice wine vinegar - .25 cup

Sesame seed oil - .5 teaspoon

Sea salt – 1 teaspoon

Garlic, minced – 1 clove

Peanut butter, natural – 2 tablespoons

Extra virgin olive oil – 2 tablespoons

Tamari sauce – 2 tablespoons

Ginger, peeled and grated – 2 teaspoons

Honey – 2 teaspoons

Black pepper, ground - .25 teaspoon

Directions

In a large salad bowl, toss together the vegetables, cilantro, and peanuts.

In a smaller bowl, whisk together the remaining ingredients until emulsified. Pour this dressing over the vegetables and toss together until fully coated.

Chill the slaw for at least ten minutes so that the flavors meld. Refrigerate the Asian slaw for up to a day in advance for deeper feelings.

Nutrition:

Calories 179

Total fat 11.8 g.

Saturated fat Trace 2.9 g.

Trans fat 0 g.

Monounsaturated fat 4.3 g.

Cholesterol Trace. 3.3 mg

Day 5 - Egg Fried Buckwheat

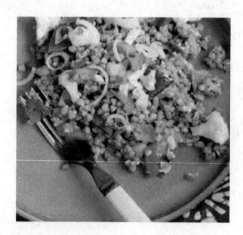

Preparation Time: 5 Minutes

Cooking time: 45 Minutes

Servings: 2

Ingredients:

Eggs, beaten – 2

Extra virgin olive oil – 2 tablespoons, divided

Onion, diced – 1

Peas, frozen - .5 cup

Carrots, finely diced – 2

Garlic, minced – 2 cloves

Ginger, grated – 1 teaspoon

Green onions, thinly sliced – 2

Tamari sauce – 2 tablespoons

Sriracha sauce – 2 teaspoons

Cooked buckwheat groats, cold – 3 cups

Directions

Add half of the olive oil to a large skillet or wok set to medium heat and add in the egg, constantly stirring until it is fully cooked. Remove the egg and transfer it to another dish.

Add the remaining olive oil to your wok along with the peas, carrots, and onion. Cook until the carrots and onions are softened, about four minutes. Add in the grated ginger and minced garlic, cooking for an additional minute until fragrant.

Add the sriracha sauce, tamari sauce, and cooked buckwheat groats to the wok. Continue to cook the buckwheat groats and stir the mixture until the buckwheat is warmed all the way through and the flavors have melded about two minutes.

Add the cooked eggs and green onions to the wok, giving it a good toss to combine and serve warm.

Nutrition:

5.68 g of protein.

1.04 g of fat.

33.5 g of carbohydrate.

4.5 g of fiber.

148 milligrams (mg) of potassium.

118 mg of phosphorus.

86 mg of magnesium.

12 mg of calcium.

Day 6 - Aromatic Ginger Turmeric Buckwheat

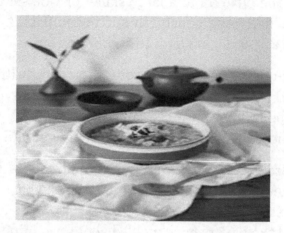

Preparation Time: 5 Minutes

Cooking time: 65 Minutes

Servings: 2

Ingredients:

Buckwheat groats rinsed and drained – 1 cup

Water – 1.75 cup

Extra virgin olive oil – 1 tablespoon

Ginger, grated – 1 tablespoon

Garlic, minced – 3 cloves

Turmeric root, grated – 1 teaspoon

Lemon juice – 1 tablespoon

Sea salt – 1 teaspoon

Cranberries, dried - .5 cup

Parsley, chopped - .33 cup

Pine nuts, toasted - .25 cup (optional)

Directions

Into a medium saucepan, add the buckwheat groats, water, olive oil, ginger, garlic, turmeric, lemon juice, and sea salt. Bring the water in the pot to a boil and then cover the mixture with a lid. Allow it to simmer over medium-low until all of the liquid is absorbed, about twenty minutes.

About fifteen minutes into the cooking time of the buckwheat sir, the dried cranberries into the buckwheat allow them to plump up the last few minutes of the cooking time.

Top the buckwheat with the pine nuts and parsley before serving.

Nutrition:

Calories 37

Day 7 - Kale and Corn Succotash

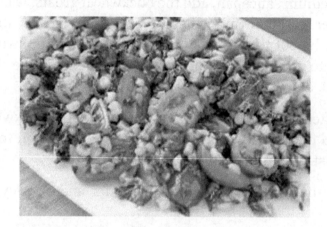

Preparation Time: 5 Minutes

Cooking time: 55 Minutes

Servings: 2

Ingredients:

Corn kernels – 2 cups

Black pepper, ground - .5 teaspoon

Kale, chopped – 2 cups

Red onion, finely diced – 1

Garlic, minced – 2 cloves

Grape tomatoes, sliced in half lengthwise – 1 cup

Sea salt – 1 teaspoon

Parsley, chopped – 2 tablespoons

Extra virgin olive oil – 1 tablespoon

Directions

Into a large skillet pour the olive oil, red onion, and the corn kernels, sauteing until hot and tender, about four minutes.

Add the sea salt, garlic, kale, and black pepper to the skillet, cooking until the kale has wilted, about three to five minutes.

Remove the large skillet from the stove and toss in the parsley and fresh grape tomatoes. Serve warm.

Nutrition:

Calories 137.4.

Total fat 6.7 g.

Saturated fat Trace 1.0 g.

Trans fat 0 g.

Monounsaturated fat 1.8 g.

Cholesterol Trace. 0.0 mg

Chapter 13: After the Diet

The two phases of the diet can be repeated as often as required for further weight loss. Also, it is recommended that you continue to add sirtfood dishes to your diet even after returning to your healthy diet. It is also recommended that you continue to drink Sirtfood juice every day. Thus, the Sirtfood diet is more like a lifestyle change than a short-term diet.

Is Sirtfood Diet Effective?

The authors of the diet make the most daring statements about this. The problem is that there is not enough evidence to support their words. There is still no convincing evidence that the Sirtfood diet helps you lose weight more effectively than any other calorie-restricted diet.

Although many of the recommended foods are undoubtedly useful, there have not been any long-term studies in humans that can confirm that overall, such a diet provides tangible health benefits. The original Sirtfood Diet book presents the results of a pilot study conducted by the authors, in which 39 volunteers from the fitness center participated. During the week, participants followed a diet and trained daily. Towards its end, they lost an average of 3.2 kg and retained or even gained muscle mass. But these results are unlikely to surprise anyone. Limiting food intake to 1000 calories a day while doing sports always leads to weight loss. The fact is that when the body is deprived of energy, it uses its reserves, in particular glycogen, in addition to burning fat and muscles. Each glycogen molecule binds 3-4 water molecules in the body. When the body uses glycogen, it also disposes of this water. As a result, we quickly lose weight, but not at the expense of fat.

Safety and side effects

Although the first stage of the Sirtfood diet contains very few calories and is an inadequate diet, given the short duration of the diet, it is unlikely to be dangerous for an average healthy adult. However, in people with diabetes, calorie restriction, and eating copious amounts of juice during the first few days can cause dangerous spikes in blood sugar levels.

Also, you are likely to feel severe hunger for all three weeks because of the low-calorie content and low fiber content in your diet. During the first phase, you may even encounter side effects such as increased fatigue and irritability.

Tips for people who decide to lose weight

Health comes first; for this reason, we should not put it into play when losing weight. It is not about eating little but learning to eat well. A healthy, varied, and complete diet includes the consumption of all types of food and is the only way to achieve a gradual, healthy, and long-term weight loss.

It is essential to incorporate physical activity into daily life progressively (walk with friends, climb stairs, go dancing), everything goes!

Weight Watchers, as an organization that focuses it, works on the dissemination of good eating habits, offers the support and follow-up necessary to help people achieve their healthy weight, and maintain it.

Basic calorie requirement

In this case, you are overweight; it is now to reduce this excess weight. First of all, you need your essential calorie needs to have a fundamental value for your project "How do I decrease the fastest?" The essential requirement is the number of calories your body consumes on average in one day. To determine your basic needs, please use our basic requirements calculator.

Only if you reduce your calorie intake slowly and allow your specific body periods of habituation, you will achieve long-term success. Your first goal now is to change your eating habits to meet your basic needs. First of all, adjust your daily calorie intake to your basic needs to avoid gaining weight. Get used to your metabolism to reduce calorie intake by keeping the daily intake of calories at the level of your basic needs for about two to three weeks.

The phase of three to four weeks. Other ways to reduce weight

If you have reached the limit to which you can reduce your calorie intake, you have already come closer to your desired weight. Therefore we come here to another method to reduce your weight.

Double is better! Do not just focus on reducing your calorie intake, but also increase your calorie needs!

In addition to reducing calorie intake, you can also increase your basic daily needs. It also depends on your daily activities. The more exercise, the more calories your body demands. If these quantities aren't delivered, your organism gets the necessary nutrients from your fat reserves. Thus, increasing your activities will contribute to a faster reduction of your fat reserves, and they will make another significant contribution to your project "How do I quickly lose weight?"

Bring movement into your life!

Every movement consumes calories. No matter what you do, the moment you make an effort, you increase your calorie consumption. You can climb stairs, ride a bike or swim, whatever you enjoy. The more movement, the faster you reach your destination!

Let your muscles play!

Your muscles are the ultimate incinerator for your excess calories. Once your muscles kick in, they need energy. And you derive that energy from burning your calories. Of course, it costs many people first to overcome some real fitness program, but once the inner bastard is overwhelmed, then the pounds fall all the faster.

Tip: With a bit of sport, you not only support your project, "How do I remove the fastest?" You also promote your health and well-being, as well as improve your quality of life.

Arm yourself against food cravings!

Food cravings are deceitful and usually hit those affected unexpectedly. You are a real threat to your project "How do I quickly lose weight?" But you can protect yourself. Helpful is a pot of tea or a walk. Even foods that keep you full longer are recommendable. Keep your blood sugar level at a low level, reducing the risk of food cravings. In case of a strong feeling of hunger, nibbling on low-calorie vegetables is often a rescue. Carrots, for example, fill your stomach but not your fat reserves.

Take your time while eating!

Whenever you take in a meal, your body needs about ten minutes to send the saturation signal, so if you eat fast, you run the risk of missing the saturation point and overeating. Therefore, ensure you eat gently and stop when full, even if something is still on the plate.

Prohibitions are wrong!

If you ask yourself, "How do I lose weight fast?" It also tends to ban certain foods. It is a wrong approach because a ban is a punishment. So if you break your ban at some point, it will cause frustration and be demotivating. You can try to do it the other way around; rewarding yourself with a small portion of what is forbidden (for example, reaching a milestone) will be positive and motivating.

Rewards generally produce better results than prohibitions and punishments. Keep your positive thinking, and do not harm your motivation by bans.

Avoid frustration!

Everyone experiences a day when everything goes wrong, and nothing works as it should. And many people try to compensate for these negative feelings with sumptuous meals. It should be avoidable. If you engage in frustration, you will quickly enter a vicious circle. You are violating your weight loss plan, causing failure and eating again. Stop this by raising your spirits and fighting stress through other centers.

How to Develop Mindful Eating Practice

The transition to the New Year is usually a time when we commit to changing something of ourselves. In these holidays, it is easy for our relationship with food to be more critical and conflicting. These are moments of "good" purposes such as "dieting," losing weight, or leaving something that causes us suffering.

However, dieting is not one of those functional purposes. It cannot be considered a skillful intention to make war on kilos or take certain foods to jail because they are guilty of our suffering.

We know that diets are not the right way to tackle problems; a path that supposes a restriction of food for our body is a form of violence that does not usually end well. Experience tells us that constraints stimulate desire, that prohibitions can only be maintained with an effort that generates excellent resistance. This resistance is directly proportional to all the energy and control that we are accumulating. There comes a time when all that effort made is of such magnitude that resistance becomes an avalanche of desire that overflows us and leads us to eat compulsively and in greater quantity.

The evidence tells us that treatments for obesity that are based on a restrictive eating plan fail in the long term, have significant adverse effects in terms of self-esteem and health. And on the other hand, we also know that dieting is the most important predictor of an eating disorder's appearance. The earlier the age at which a person begins dieting, the more risk he has of developing an eating disorder.

That is why it is essential to focus on a change in our relationship with food and reorient our relationship with it from a perspective of compassion, generosity, and forgiveness.

Eating mindfully is a perspective that allows us to approach difficulties from kindness, acceptance, and lack of judgment is a radical change that will enable us to open ourselves to new ways of relating to our problems, with food and with life in general.

Eating with mindful attention or mindful eating has been described by Jan Chozen Bays as "... an experience that involves body, mind, heart, and spirit to choose, prepare and eat food." It allows us to be curious to investigate our responses to food and food. Our inner signals of hunger and satiety and nurture ourselves by listening to the wisdom of our bodies. In this way, mindful eating allows us to make choices that promote health and well-being.

From the perspective of mindful eating, the idea of labeling food as "good" or "bad" is abandoned, calories are not counted, diets are not prescribed, and it is not said what "should" or "should not be" eaten or prohibited or restricted foods. Instead, awareness of the internal signs of hunger and satiety is cultivated, and the wisdom of our body begins to be rediscovered.

Conclusion

Throughout this book, you have learned how the Sirt diet is much more than a weight loss plan for celebrities. While yes, it may work for stars, it can help anyone reach their weight loss goals. You can enjoy delicious meals, nutritious ingredients, a variety of health benefits, and functional and maintainable weight loss. Whether you choose to practice the traditional or natural approach to the Sirt diet, you will find that you can lose weight with a simple and straightforward approach.

Please remember that this book is not making medical claims or offering medical advice; you should always speak to your doctor about changes in your diet and exercise. However, studies have shown many health benefits can be attained from eating the polyphenols found in Sirtfoods. These studies indicate that not only can these foods increase weight loss, they can also treat some of the most common ailments in our modern age—such as diabetes, heart disease, stroke, and more. While there may be few studies on the Sirt diet at this time, studies on caloric restriction and Sirt Foods are clear: there are many benefits.

5 truth practically everybody makes Sirtfood diet

1. Eating foods that you cannot actually like

In case you believe you are going to turn into a fan of Brussels sprouts as it's January second and you've not eaten anything in the last 3 months weeks, you are setting yourself up to fail. One explanation diets do not work: they induce people to eat things that they don't like. "If the carrot smoothie isn't exercising for you, take sautéed lettuce, celery, tofu chips. Better, ditch the carrot and attempt lettuce, collard greens, Swiss chard, or still another vegetable" the following secret to eating healthy without quitting life would be really to test out spices. "Do not forget to take in various seasonings or manners of cooking. By way of instance, get a Cajun spice combination or five-spice and scatter it together with one's poultry or veggies.

2. Expecting immediate results

The observing you did on Christmas isn't going to become reversed following weekly. The most straightforward way to fall short of one's resolution or goal is to help it become unattainable. For example, resolving to prevent you from eating your favorite takeout food or planning to lose 10 lbs within 1 month may backfire. That is not because allowing the foods that you like results in finally bingeing to them once you cannot tolerate the craving. And seeking to reduce a lot of weight too fast will undoubtedly cause disappointment.

The key would be to put smaller goals that build up to an objective, he states. This means that you may attempt to prevent this take out joint more frequently than you can today or wish to lose a couple of pounds weekly --and soon you finally reach your target," she states.

3. Maybe not getting meals in front of time

One of the reasons people overeat around Christmas is that there is a large amount of food outside; it is easy to catch. Whenever the observing is finished, make it simple to choose healthful options by organizing healthy food beforehand. It is possible to arrive at it when you are hungry, rather than earning a game-time decision when you are mesmerized. Meal preparation is critical to eating a balanced diet program. Cut vegetables up and also make additional portions of dinner to the week beforehand. In this manner, it is possible to collect dinner very quickly for a busy week.

Now you won't think some of the strangest things a few individuals did to eliminate weight:

4. Maybe not assessing labels at the supermarket

Being a little more particular regarding the foods that you buy at the store will be able to assist you in getting right back on the right track without any difficulty. Examine the food labels to the ingredients before you buy something. That will produce a more informed decision regarding whether it belongs in what you eat plan. Chen says it mainly crucial to pay careful attention to serving sizes. "A jar of juice might comprise two portions," she states. This means it includes twice the calories and sugar just as what's recorded on the tag. And as you are not likely in the habit of just drinking half a juice, then which will prevent you from losing weight. Other critical elements to consider will be the total amount of protein and fiber in meals. Take 2 g of fiber and 20 g of protein into every meal to remain full and fulfilled.

5. Maybe not acquiring a backup policy for seconds weakness

Putting a strategy set up to modify your daily diet is fantastic. However, you've also must have a policy for roadblocks. Simply take stress eating throughout a mainly annoying afternoon, such as. Once you learn, you are enticed to make yourself feel a lot better with the assistance of ice cream, then look for a backup program. Maybe you opt to find yourself a 20-minute massage at a nail salon or blow some steam off from the particular candlelight yoga class. Both are welcome adjustments to a healthier new way of life, and you'll feel far better in the long term.

Why a Balanced Diet Is Your Key to Success

Far too often, one hears beginners in the gym complain that they could eat now since their diet has been changed, nothing more. This usually ends in simplicity with a classic bodybuilder diet of rice and turkey. Of course, you won't be able to live with this in the long run and live happily.

You will learn how to balance your diet so as not to lose the fun of eating. This will make it easier for you to change permanently.

Versatility Makes the Difference

Since only the calories and the macronutrient distribution play a decisive role in the diet, many foods lead to the desired goal.

However, you should pay attention to what macronutrients you take because carbohydrates are not equal to carbohydrates!

It is also vital for our health to look for a varied and balanced diet. Only in this way is the absorption of all substances necessary for the body ensured.

The Length Matters!

As mentioned earlier, carbohydrates are not equal to carbohydrates. As every child knows, both simple sugars and starches are "saccharides." However, they have various effects on the body.

Our body can only use sugar in the form of glucose, that is, simple sugars. Since starch consists of many glucose molecules, it must first be "decomposed" by the body. This process takes time, which is why glucose is released successively.

If we eat high-glucose foods, the pure sugar in the blood rises very quickly and slowly because nothing has to be processed. After all, starchy foods provide energy for a long time and glucose-containing meals only for a short time.

As a result, you should eat short-chain carbohydrates before and after training, and otherwise long-chain ones.

Good sources:

- Short-chain carbohydrates:
- Honey
- Fruit (bananas etc.)

- Energy bar
- Dark chocolate

Long-chain carbohydrates:

Sweet potatoes or potatoes

- Rice
- Noodles
- Beans, peas, etc.
- Whole grain bread

Do Not Be Afraid Of Fats!

Like carbohydrates, many laypeople are afraid of fats. This fear is, of course, unfounded and relies on many myths. Fats are an essential building material of our bodies.

For example, fats play a decisive role in the transmission of stimuli and regulate our hormone balance. Every athlete knows how outstanding the hormone balance is for muscle building and athletic success. Therefore, it can have fatal consequences to avoid fats in principle.

As with carbohydrates, you have to differentiate with the fats. One distinguishes between saturated and unsaturated fatty acids. Often the saturated fatty acids are considered the "bad guys." But what is there?

Do saturated fatty acids lead to a heart attack?

Several studies are showing that saturated fat increases cholesterol and causes heart attacks. Again and again, however, new studies question precisely this. The statement that saturated fatty acids are unhealthy cannot, therefore, be supported on a flat-rate basis.

If you have a micronutrient-rich diet and enough exercise, you do not have to worry about saturated fat as part of your calorie balance.

Monounsaturated fatty acids

Monounsaturated fatty acids are not a problem for your health as part of a balanced diet. Like all other fats, they serve as an energy source.

One finds the monounsaturated fatty acids, for example, in olive oil. The problem is only the Trans fats; these are very common in industrially hardened fats. These should be avoided at all costs and should not be consumed too often as they can be problematic for our health.

Polyunsaturated fatty acids / essential fatty acids

Essential fatty acids belong to the group that your body can not produce itself. So he depends on you feeding her from outside.

The essential fatty acids are among the unsaturated fatty acids. One distinguishes between:

Omega 3

Omega 6

A good source of omega 3 is greasy fish, such as herring, tuna, or salmon.

Vegan sources are linseed oil, hemp oil, walnut oil. These oils should not be utilized for cooking and should, therefore, be used only cold. Also, chia seeds are a good omega 3 source and are also beneficial for our gut health.

Most of the time, Omega 6 is absorbed enough by the daily diet. It, therefore, makes sense to supplement Omega 3 to prevent an imbalance. Ideally, the ratio of Omega 6 to Omega 3 should be between 1: 1 and 5: 1.

So, what are you waiting for? The sooner you begin, the sooner you can reach your goals. You have everything you need to reach for and grab hold of the success you desire. All you have to do is take the first step